Lisa G. Torres.

OPTAVIA DIET COOKBOOK

Start Your Lifelong Transformation With 250 Quick and Easy Recipes. Make Your Body and Your Mind Happy Without Overthinking Meal Preparation

© Copyright 2020 - All rights reserved.

Table of Contents

Introduction

If you are looking to lose weight fast and you don't always have enough time to cook, OPTAVIA is the best option for you. However, the OPTAVIA program requires that you work with a coach on a one-on-one guide and counseling. It includes branded products known as Fuelings and homemade food known as Lean & Green meals.

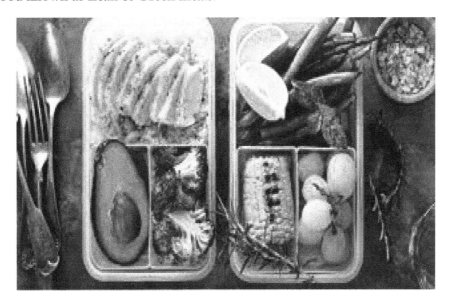

These Fuelings have over 60 products that are low in carb and high in protein. They have probiotic cultures with health-promoting bacteria that boost gut health. Some of them are bars, shakes, cereals, cookies, pasta, puddings, etc.

The Diet Programs

The OPTAVIA program has three versions, which include 2 weight loss plans and a maintenance plan.

- **Optimal Weight 5&1**: This plan is the most popular among the program plans. It is made up of daily 5 Fuelings and 1 lean and green meal.

- **Optimal Weight 4&2&1**: If you need more calories, this plan is for you. It is more flexible and includes 4 Fuelings, 2 lean and green, and 1 snack every day.

- **Optimal Health 3&3**: With 3 Fuelings and 3 lean and green meals, it is designed to help in weight maintenance.

Optavia Diet Guide

For a quick weight loss goal, the Optimal Weight 5&1 Plan may be the best plan to start with. Most people with the target of losing weight usually go for this plan as it helps them to drop up to 12 pounds within 12 weeks.

In the Optimal Weight 5&1 Plan, you are expected to eat one lean and green meal and five OPTAVIA Fuelings. These meals are to be eaten every 2-3 hours intervals. Then, you will back it up with 30 minutes of exercise. Your coach will direct you on the best approach.

However, the daily carbs from meals and Fuelings should not exceed 100 grams. You can get meals and Fuelings from the company. Though it may not be cost-effective, this book is designed to help you save costs. You can prepare the meals by yourself to reduce costs.

There are a plethora of recipes in this book to help you along the process for your daily meals. You can also eat out, but keep in mind that you must follow the diet plan as instructed by your coach. However, alcohol is highly restricted for this plan.

Once you get to your desired weight, you are expected to enter the maintenance phase. This is a transition phase that requires a gradual increase in your daily calorie intake to no more than 1,550 cal. You can add a wider variety of food to your daily meals, which include fruits, whole grains, and low-fat dairy.

The maintenance phase is expected to last for 6 weeks before you move to the Optimal Health 3&3 Plan. In this plan, your daily food intake will be 3 OPTAVIA Fuelings and 3 lean and green meals.

In the OPTAVIA diet, most people that follow the diet usually opt for the 5&1 plan. The 5&1 program is made up of 5 Fuelings and 1 high protein low-carb meal. There are over 60 fueling options in the OPTAVIA diet, and these options include bars, puddings, shakes, soups, biscuits, etc. These Fuelings contain probiotics that help to promote digestive health.

The interesting aspect of the OPTAVIA diet is its flexibility, which makes it easier to work with. Once you reach your desired weight goal, you can easily switch to the 3&3 plan. Transitioning to this weight-maintenance plan is easy since you have already changed the old unhealthy eating habits. For those looking to consume more calories, the 4&2&1 plan is your best bet. With the 4&2&1 plan, you take 4 Fuelings, 2 healthy lean and green meals, and 1 snack.

How OPTAVIA Can Help You Lose Weight

How much weight you lose on the OPTAVIA diet depends mostly on how active and how you follow the plan. If you stick with the plan and stay very active, you will lose more weight. Many have tried it, and it worked perfectly well. The following research studies show how effective the OPTAVIA diet can be when strictly followed. Though the research is mostly on Medifast, OPTAVIA and Medifast have identical macro-nutrients and can be interchanged to achieve the same result. So, the studies are valid for both OPTAVIA and Medifast plans.

- A study published in the Obesity journal in 2016 showed that after 12 weeks of observing the Medifast (OPTAVIA) diet guide, obese people lost 8.8% body weight.

- The study released by John Hopkins Medicine that ran for 12 weeks revealed that weight-loss programs like Medifast are effective for a long-term weight loss goal.

- A study in the Nutrition Journal carried out in 2015 shows that 310 obese and overweight people who followed the Medifast (OPTAVIA) diet plan lost 24 lb in 12 weeks. In the 24th week, the average weight loss recorded was 35 lb.

- Another study published in the Nutrition Journal shows that 90 obese adults who followed the 5&1 plan lost an average of 30 pounds in 16 weeks.

- The analysis published in the Eating and Weight Disorder Journal in 2008 shows that the average weight loss recorded on 324 obese patients in 12 weeks was 21 lb and 26 ½ lb after 24 weeks. However, these patients also took appetite suppressant.

Is OPTAVIA Diet Easy To Follow?

If you are someone like me that likes trying so many treats and yummy recipes almost every day, the OPTAVIA diet may not be easy in the long term. However, the OPTAVIA diet is programmed to accommodate both long-term and short-term goals. There are three major diet plans to choose from to suit your desired eating habit.

The 5&1 plan may not be easy in the long-term, but there are over 60 fueling options to work with. Moreover, you have a plethora of resources where you can get recipes, including this cookbook with so many mouthwatering recipes to make.

Unlike most weight-loss diets, you don't need to stress yourself counting calories, points, or carbs. Though they are needed for reference purposes, you don't need to kill yourself over it as long as the meals you are taking are OPTAVIA-compliance lean and green meals.

Interestingly, you can easily eat out while on the OPTAVIA diet. The main thing is for you to understand the guidelines and follow them judiciously. You can as well download the eating out guide from the company website to help you easily navigate the buffets and eateries.

How Much Exercise Is Needed?

Like we stated earlier, if you want to lose weight as desired, you need to be active. Exercise helps you achieve that. Find the right exercise you can easily do on a daily basis and incorporate it into your plan.

OPTAVIA highly recommends at least 30 minutes of exercise almost every day. If it's walking, walk. If it requires doing some minor workouts, do them and enjoy the process. Remember, happiness is of the utmost importance in your daily life. So, engage in the exercise that you enjoy most and are super healthy for you. Don't overstress your body, don't go overboard. You can get recommendations from your doctor or coach if you have any.

CHAPTER 1:

What to Eat

Best Foods for OPTAVIA Diet

Your homemade meals are expected to be mostly low-carb vegetables, lean proteins, and a few healthy fats. Low-carb beverages such as coffee, water, tea, unsweetened almond milk, etc, are allowed, but in small amounts.

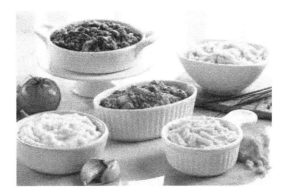

- The recommended foods for your lean and green meals are;

- Fish and Shellfish: trout, halibut, salmon, shrimp, tuna, crab, lobster, scallops.

- Meat: Lean beef, pork chop, tenderloin, turkey, chicken, lamb.

- Eggs: egg whites, whole eggs, and egg beaters.

- Soy: tofu

- Oil: vegetable oils - flaxseed, olive, canola, walnut, lemon oil, etc

- Fats: avocado, olives, almonds, pistachios, reduced-fat margarine, walnuts, etc.

- Vegetables: zucchini, cauliflower, celery, mushrooms, eggplant, pepper, spinach, cucumbers, squash, broccoli, collard, jicama, etc.

- Snacks (sugar-free): mints, popsicle, gum, gelatin, etc.

- Beverages (sugar-free): coffee, water, tea, almond milk, etc.

- Seasoning and condiments: spices, dried herbs, salsa, cocktail sauce, yellow mustard, lemon juice, soy sauce, lime juice, etc.

Avoid These Foods

Except for the carbs in the Fuelings, the OPTAVIA diet restricts most foods and beverages with carb content. Some fats are not allowed, including fried foods. Avoid the following foods in your daily meals;

- Refined grains: including pasta, flour tortillas, cookies, white rice, white bread, cakes, biscuits, etc.

- Whole fat dairy: including yogurt, milk, and cheese.

- Fried foods: including fish, veggies, meats, pastries, etc.

- Fats: like coconut oil, butter, etc.

- Alcohol: all types.

- Beverages: like an energy drink, fruit juice, sweet tea, soda, etc

If you are on the 5&1 plan, you need to avoid the following foods in your daily meal. You can introduce them in the transition phase;

- Starchy veggies: white potatoes, sweet potatoes, peas, and corn.

- Whole grains: brown rice, whole grain bread, whole-wheat pasta, etc.

- Low-fat dairy: cheese, yogurt, and milk.

- Legumes: beans, peas, soybeans, lentils, etc.

- Fruits: fresh fruits. Eat more berries when you enter the transition phase.

CHAPTER 2:

Lean and Green Recipes

Chicken Salad

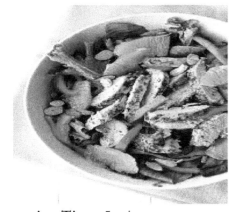

Preparation Time: 5 minutes

Cooking Time: 25 minutes

Servings: 4

Ingredients:

For Chicken:

- 1 ¾ lb. boneless, skinless chicken breast
- ¼ teaspoon each of pepper and salt (or as desired)
- 1 ½ tablespoon of butter, melted

For Mediterranean salad:

- 1 cup of sliced cucumber
- 6 cups of romaine lettuce that is torn or roughly chopped
- 10 pitted Kalamata olives
- 1 pint of cherry tomatoes
- 1/3 cup of reduced-fat feta cheese
- ¼ teaspoon each of pepper and salt (or lesser)
- 1 small lemon juice (it should be about 2 tablespoons)

Directions:

1. Preheat your oven or grill to about 350°F. Season the chicken with salt, butter, and black pepper
2. Roast or grill chicken until it reaches an internal temperature of 165°F in about 25 minutes. Once your chicken breasts are cooked, remove and keep aside to rest for about 5 minutes before you slice it. Combine all the salad ingredients you have and toss everything together very well. Serve the chicken with Mediterranean salad

Nutrition: Calories 340, Fat 4, Carbs 9, Protein 45

Chipotle Chicken & Cauliflower Rice Bowls

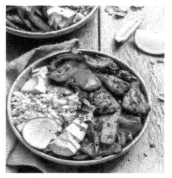

Preparation Time: 10 minutes

Cooking Time: 20 minutes

Servings: 4

Ingredients: 1/3 cup of salsa - 1 quantity of 14.5 oz. of can fire-roasted diced tomatoes

- 1 canned chipotle pepper + 1 teaspoon sauce - ½ teaspoon of dried oregano
- 1 teaspoon of cumin

- 1 ½ lb. of boneless, skinless chicken breast - ¼ teaspoon of salt
- 1 cup of reduced-fat shredded Mexican cheese blend
- 4 cups of frozen riced cauliflower
- ½ medium-sized avocado, sliced

Directions:

1. Combine the first ingredients in a blender and blend until they become smooth. Place chicken inside your instant pot, and pour the sauce over it. Cover the lid and close the pressure valve. Set it to 20 minutes at high temperature. Let the pressure release on its own before opening. Remove the piece and the chicken, and then add it back to the sauce. Microwave the riced cauliflower according to the directions on the package
2. Before you serve, divide the riced cauliflower, cheese, avocado, and chicken equally among the 4 bowls.

Nutrition: Calories 276, Fat 12, Carbs 19, Protein 35

Lemon Garlic Oregano Chicken with Asparagus

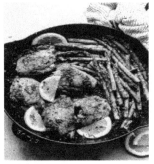

Preparation Time: 5 minutes
Cooking Time: 40 minutes
Servings: 4
Ingredients:

- 1 small lemon, juiced (this should be about 2 tablespoons of lemon juice)

- 1 ¾ lb. of bone-in, skinless chicken thighs - 2 tablespoon of fresh oregano, minced - 2 cloves of garlic, minced
- 2 lbs. of asparagus, trimmed
- ¼ teaspoon each or less for black pepper and salt

Directions:

1. Preheat the oven to about 350°F.
2. Put the chicken in a medium-sized bowl. Now, add the garlic, oregano, lemon juice, pepper, and salt and toss together to combine. Roast the chicken in the air fryer oven until it reaches an internal temperature of 165°F in about 40 minutes. Once the chicken thighs have been cooked, remove and keep aside to rest. Now, steam the asparagus on a stovetop or in a microwave to the desired doneness. Serve asparagus with the roasted chicken thighs.

Nutrition: Calories 356, Fat 10, Carbs 10, Protein 24

Sheet Pan Chicken Fajita Lettuce Wraps

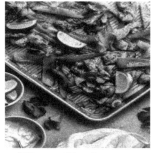

Preparation Time: 15 minutes
Cooking Time: 30 minutes
Servings: 2
Ingredients:

- 1 lb. chicken breast, thinly sliced into strips
- 2 teaspoon of olive oil
- 2 bell peppers, thinly sliced into strips
- 2 teaspoon of fajita seasoning
- 6 leaves from a romaine heart

- Juice of half a lime
- ¼ cup plain of non-fat Greek yogurt

Directions:

1. Preheat your oven to about 400°F
2. Combine all of the ingredients except for lettuce in a large plastic bag that can be resealed. Mix very well to coat vegetables and chicken with oil and seasoning evenly.
3. Spread the contents of the bag evenly on a foil-lined baking sheet. Bake it for about25-30 minutes, until the chicken is thoroughly cooked.
4. Serve on lettuce leaves and topped with Greek yogurt if you like

Nutrition: Calories 387, Fat 6, Carbs 14, Protein 18

Savory Cilantro Salmon

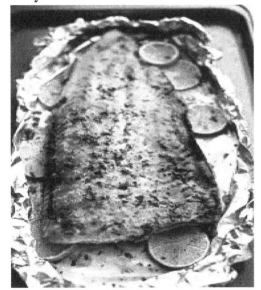

Preparation Time: 10 minutes
Cooking Time: 30 minutes
Servings: 4
Ingredients:

- 2 tablespoons of fresh lime or lemon
- 4 cups of fresh cilantro, divided
- 2 tablespoon of hot red pepper sauce
- ½ teaspoon of salt. Divided

- 1 teaspoon of cumin
- 4, 7 oz. of salmon filets
- ½ cup of (4 oz.) water
- 2 cups of sliced red bell pepper
- 2 cups of sliced yellow bell pepper
- 2 cups of sliced green bell pepper
- Cooking spray
- ½ teaspoon of pepper

Directions:

1. Get a blender or food processor and combine half of the cilantro, lime juice or lemon, cumin, hot red pepper sauce, water, and salt; then puree until they become smooth. Transfer the marinade gotten into a large re-sealable plastic bag.
2. Add salmon to marinade. Seal the bag, squeeze out air that might have been trapped inside, turn to coat salmon. Refrigerate for about 1 hour, turning as often as possible.
3. Now, after marinating, preheat your oven to about 400°F. Arrange the pepper slices in a single layer in a slightly-greased, medium-sized square baking dish. Bake it for 20 minutes, turn the pepper slices once.
4. Drain your salmon and do away with the marinade. Crust the upper part of the salmon with the remaining chopped, fresh cilantro.
5. Place salmon on the top of the pepper slices and bake for about 12-14 minutes until you observe that the fish flakes easily when it is being tested with a fork
6. Enjoy

Nutrition: Calories 350, Fat 13, Carbs 15, Protein 42

Lean and Green "Macaroni"

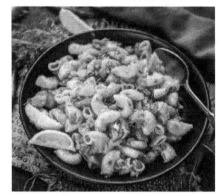

Preparation Time: 10 minutes

Cooking Time: 30 minutes

Servings: 2

Ingredients

- 2 tablespoons yellow onion, diced
- 5 ounces 95-97% lean ground beef
- 2 tablespoons light thousand island dressing
- 1/8 teaspoon apple cider vinegar
- 1/8 teaspoon onion powder
- 3 cups Romaine lettuce, shredded
- 2 tablespoons low-fat cheddar cheese, shredded
- 1-ounce dill pickle slices
- 1 teaspoon sesame seeds

Directions:

1. Put 3 tablespoons of water in a pan and heat over medium-low flame. Water sauté the onions for 30 seconds before adding the beef. Sauté the beef for 4 minutes while stirring constantly.
2. Add in the thousand island dressing, apple cider vinegar, and onion powder. Close the lid and keep on cooking for 5 minutes. Remove the lid and allow to simmer until the sauce thickens. Turn off the heat and allow the beef to rest and cool.
3. In a bowl, place the lettuce at the bottom and pour in the beef. Layer with cheddar cheese and pickles. Sprinkle with sesame on top.

Nutrition: Calories 412, Fat 8, Carbs 18, Protein 4

Lean and Green Broccoli Taco

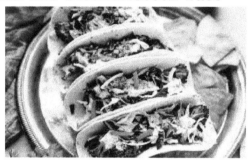

Preparation Time: 10 minutes

Cooking Time: 15 minutes

Servings: 2

Ingredients:

- 4 ounces 95-97% lean ground beef
- ¼ cup roma tomatoes, chopped
- ¼ teaspoon garlic powder
- ¼ teaspoon onion powder
- 1 ¼ cup broccoli, cut into bite-sized pieces
- A pinch of red pepper flakes
- 1 ounce low-sodium cheddar cheese, shredded

Directions:

1. Place 3 tablespoons of water in a pan and heat over medium flame. Water sauté the beef and tomatoes for 5 minutes until the tomatoes are wilted. Add in the garlic and onion powder and stir for another 3 minutes.
2. Add the broccoli and close the lid. Cook for another 5 minutes.
3. Garnish with red pepper flakes and cheddar cheese on top.

Nutrition: Calories 412, Fat 6, Carbs 20, Protein 6

Lean and Green Crunchy Chicken Tacos

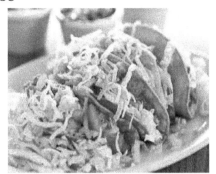

Preparation Time: 10 minutes
Cooking Time: 10 minutes
Servings: 2
Ingredients:

- ½ cup low sodium chicken stock
- 2 chicken breasts, minced
- 1 red onion, chopped
- 1 clove of garlic, minced
- 3 plum tomatoes, chopped
- 1 teaspoon cumin powder
- 1 teaspoon cinnamon powder
- 1 teaspoon ground coriander
- 1 red onion, chopped
- ½ red chili, chopped
- 1 tablespoon lime juice
- Meat from 1 ripe avocado
- 1 cucumber, sliced into thick rounds

Directions:

1. Place a tablespoon of chicken stock in a pan and heat over medium flame. Water sauté the chicken, onion, garlic, and tomatoes for 4 minutes or until the tomatoes have wilted.
2. Season with cumin, cinnamon, and coriander. Reduce the heat to low and cook for another 5 minutes. Set aside and allow to cool.
3. In a bowl, mix together the onion, chili, lime juice, and mashed avocado. This is the salsa.
4. Scoop the salsa and top on sliced cucumber. Top with cooked chicken.

Nutrition: Calories 447, Fat 8, Carbs 12, Protein 24

Optavia-Approved Vegetarian Zucchini Lasagna

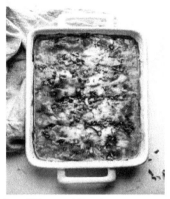

Preparation Time: 10 minutes
Cooking Time: 10 minutes
Servings: 2
Ingredients:

- 1 ¼ pounds zucchini, sliced into lasagna
- ¼ cup chopped fresh spinach
- 1 ½ cup sugar-free and low-sodium marinara sauce
- 2/3 cup mozzarella cheese, shredded
- 1 cup part-skim ricotta cheese
- Fresh basil for garnish

Directions:

1. Preheat the oven to 3750F for 5 minutes.
2. Place the zucchini slices in a dish and layer with spinach, marinara sauce, mozzarella, and ricotta cheese. Repeat the process until several layers are formed.
3. Top with basil.
4. Place in the oven and bake for 10 minutes.

Nutrition: Calories 412, Fat 9, Carbs 16, Protein 6

Lean and Green Chicken Chili

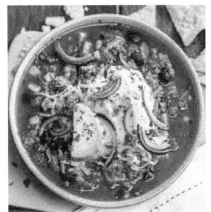

Preparation Time: 10 minutes

Cooking Time: 45 minutes

Servings: 2

Ingredients:

- 1-pound boneless skinless chicken breast, chopped
- 1 teaspoon ground cumin
- 1 cup chopped poblano pepper
- ½ cup chopped onion
- 1 clove of garlic, minced
- 2 cups low-sodium chicken broth
- 1 cup rehydrated pinto beans
- 1 cup chopped tomatoes
- 2 tablespoons minced cilantro

Directions:

1. Place all ingredients except the cilantro in a pressure cooker.
2. Close the lid and set the vent to the sealing position.
3. Cook on high for 45 minutes until the beans are soft.
4. Garnish with cilantro before serving.

Nutrition: Calories 229, Fat 12, Carbs 23, Protein 21

Avocado, Citrus, and Shrimp Salad

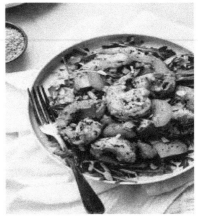

Preparation Time: 10 minutes

Cooking Time: 4 minutes

Servings: 2

Ingredients:

- 1 head green leaf lettuce
- 1 avocado
- ½ pound wild-caught shrimp
- 2 tablespoons olive oil
- Juice of 1 lemon

Directions:

1. Place the lettuce in a bowl and top with mashed avocado meat.
2. Clean the shrimps by deveining and removing the head.
3. Heat oil in a skillet over medium-low heat and heat the oil. Cook the shrimps for 2 minutes on each side.
4. Place the shrimps on top of mashed avocado and drizzle with lemon juice.

Nutrition: Calories 359, Fat 5, Carbs 16, Protein 6

Lean and Green Broccoli Alfredo

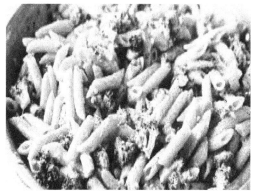

Ingredients:
Preparation Time: 10 minutes
Cooking Time: 2 minutes
Servings: 2
Ingredients:

- 2 heads of broccoli, cut into florets
- 2 tablespoons lemon juice, freshly squeezed
- ½ cup cashew, soaked for 2 hours in water then drained
- 2 tablespoons white miso, low sodium
- 2 teaspoon Dijon mustard
- Freshly cracked black pepper

Directions:
1. Boil water in a pot over medium flame. Blanch the broccoli for 2 minutes, then place in a bowl of iced water. Drain.
2. In a food processor, place the remaining ingredients and pulse until smooth.
3. Pour the alfredo sauce over the broccoli. Toss to coat with the sauce.

Nutrition: Calories 156, Fat 4, Carbs 21, Protein 4

Lean and Green Steak Machine

Preparation Time: 10 minutes
Cooking Time: 10 minutes
Servings: 4
Ingredients:

- 1/2 teaspoon extra virgin olive oil

- 2 ounces Sirloin steak, 98% lean
- Salt and pepper to taste
- 1 zucchini, cut into long thin strips
- 1 onion, chopped
- 6 ounces asparagus, blanched
- 4 ounces peas, blanched

Directions:
1. Heat olive oil in a skillet. Season the steak with salt and pepper to taste.
2. Place in the skillet and sear the steak for 5 minutes on each side. Allow to rest for five minutes before slicing into strips.
3. Place the remaining ingredients in a bowl and season with salt and pepper to taste
4. Top with steak strips, then toss to combine all ingredients.

Nutrition: Calories 174, Fat 8, Carbs 23, Protein 8

Garlic Shrimp Zucchini Noodles

Preparation Time: 10 minutes
Cooking Time: 4 minutes
Servings: 2
Ingredients:

- 16 ounces uncooked shrimps, shelled and deveined
- 1 tablespoon olive oil
- 1 cup cherry tomatoes, cut in half
- 8 cups zucchini strips
- 2 tablespoons minced garlic
- 1 teaspoon dried oregano
- ½ teaspoon chili powder
- ½ teaspoon salt

Directions:
1. Brush the shrimps with olive oil. Place on a skillet and cook for 2 minutes on all sides or until pink. Set aside.

2. Place the rest of the ingredients in a bowl and add the shrimps. Season with salt, then toss to coat the ingredients.

Nutrition: Calories 633, Fat 6, Carbs 32, Protein 12

Broccoli Kale Salmon Burgers

Preparation Time: 10 minutes
Cooking Time: 30 minutes
Servings: 2
Ingredients:

- 2 eggs
- ½ cup onion, chopped
- ½ cup broccoli, chopped
- ½ cup kale, chopped
- ½ tsp garlic powder
- 2 tbsp lemon juice
- ½ cup almond flour
- 15 oz can salmon, drained and bones removed
- ½ tsp salt

Directions:

1. Line one plate with parchment paper and set aside.
2. Add all ingredients into the large bowl and mix until well combined.
3. Make five equal shapes of patties from the mixture and place them on a prepared plate.
4. Place the plate in the refrigerator for 30 minutes.
5. Spray a large pan with cooking spray and heat over medium heat.
6. Once the pan is hot, add patties and cook for 5-7 minutes per side.
7. Serve and enjoy.

Nutrition: Calories 221, Fat 6, Carbs 18, Protein 8

Pan Seared Cod

Preparation Time: 10 minutes
Cooking Time: 25 minutes
Servings: 2
Ingredients:

- 1 ¾ lbs cod fillets
- 1 tbsp ranch seasoning
- 4 tsp olive oil

Directions:

1. Heat oil in a large pan over medium-high heat.
2. Season fish fillets with ranch seasoning.
3. Once the oil is hot, place fish fillets in a pan and cook for 6-8 minutes on each side.
4. Serve immediately and enjoy.

Nutrition: Calories 204, Fat 6, Carbs 12, Protein 6

Quick Lemon Pepper Salmon

Preparation Time: 10 minutes
Cooking Time: 18 minutes
Servings: 2
Ingredients:

- 1 ½ lbs salmon fillets
- ½ tsp ground black pepper
- 1 tsp dried oregano
- 2 garlic cloves, minced
- ¼ cup olive oil
- 1 lemon juice
- 1 tsp sea salt

Directions:

1. In a large bowl, mix together lemon juice, olive oil, garlic, oregano, black pepper, and salt.
2. Add fish fillets in bowl and coat well with the marinade, and place in the refrigerator for 15 minutes.
3. Preheat the grill.
4. Brush grill grates with oil.
5. Place marinated salmon fillets on a hot grill and cook for 4 minutes, then turn

salmon fillets to the other side and cook for 4 minutes more.

Nutrition: Calories 340, Fat 6, Carbs 31, Protein 28

Tomatillo and Green Chili Pork Stew

Preparation Time: 10 minutes

Cooking Time: 20 minutes

Servings: 4

Ingredients:

- 2 scallions, chopped
- 2 cloves of garlic
- 1 lb. tomatillos, trimmed and chopped
- 2 serrano chilies, seeds, and membranes
- ½ tsp of dried Mexican oregano (or you can use regular oregano)
- 1 ½ lb. of boneless pork loin, to be cut into bite-sized cubes
- ¼ cup of cilantro, chopped
- ¼ tablespoon (each) salt and paper
- 1 jalapeno, seeds and membranes to be removed and thinly sliced
- 1 cup of sliced radishes
- 4 lime wedges

Directions:

1. Combine all ingredients and puree until smooth
2. Season with pepper & salt, and cover it simmers. Simmer on the heat for approximately 20 minutes.

Nutrition: Calories 356, Fat 19, Carbs 11, Protein 23

Optavia Cloud Bread

Preparation Time: 25 minutes

Cooking Time: 35 minutes

Servings: 3

Ingredients:

- ½ cup of Fat-free 0% Plain Greek Yogurt (4.4 0z)

- 3 Eggs, Separated
- 16 teaspoon Cream of Tartar
- 1 Packet sweetener (a granulated sweetener just like stevia)

Directions:

1. For about 30 minutes before making this meal, place the Kitchen Aid Bowl and the whisk attachment in the freezer.
2. Preheat your oven to 30 degrees
3. Remove the mixing bowl and whisk attachment from the freezer
4. Separate the eggs. Now put the egg whites in the Kitchen Aid Bowl, and they should be in a different medium-sized bowl.
5. In the medium-sized bowl containing the yolks, mix in the sweetener and yogurt.
6. In the bowl containing the egg white, add in the cream of tartar. Beat this mixture until the egg whites turn to stiff peaks.
7. Now, take the egg yolk mixture and carefully fold it into the egg whites. Be cautious and avoid over-stirring.
8. Place baking paper on a baking tray and spray with cooking spray.
9. Scoop out 6 equally-sized "blobs" of the "dough" onto the parchment paper.
10. Bake for about 25-35 minutes (make sure you check when it is 25 minutes, in some ovens, they are done at this timestamp). You will know they are done as they will get brownish at the top and have some crack.
11. Most people like them cold against being warm
12. Most people like to re-heat in a toast oven or toaster to get them a little bit crispy.
13. Your serving size should be about 2 pieces.

Nutrition: Calories 234, Fat 4, Carbs 5, Protein 23

Avocado Lime Shrimp Salad

Preparation Time: 15 minutes

Cooking Time: 0 minutes

Servings: 2

Ingredients:

- 14 ounces of jumbo cooked shrimp, peeled and deveined; chopped
- 4 ½ ounces of avocado, diced
- 1 ½ cup of tomato, diced
- ¼ cup of chopped green onion
- ¼ cup of jalapeno with the seeds removed, diced fine
- 1 teaspoon of olive oil
- 2 tablespoons of lime juice
- 1/8 teaspoon of salt
- 1 tablespoon of chopped cilantro

Directions:

1. Get a small bowl and combine green onion, olive oil, lime juice, pepper, a pinch of salt. Wait for about 5 minutes for all of them to marinate and mellow the flavor of the onion.
2. Get a large bowl and combine chopped shrimp, tomato, avocado, jalapeno. Combine all of the ingredients, add cilantro, and gently toss.
3. Add pepper and salt as desired.

Nutrition: Calories 312, Fat 6, Carbs 15, Protein 26

CHAPTER 3:

Fuelings

Avocado Bites

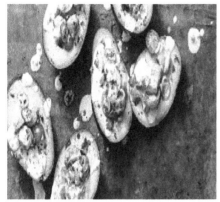

Preparation time: 10 minutes
Cooking time: 0 minutes
Servings: 2
Ingredients:

- 2 avocados, peeled, pitted, and cubed
- 2 tablespoons sweet paprika
- juice of 1 lemon 1 teaspoon basil, dried
- 1 teaspoon oregano, dried
- Salt and black pepper to the taste

Directions:

1. Mix the ingredients and serve.

Nutrition: calories 60, fat 3, carbs 4.2, protein 4.4

Chives Dip

Preparation time: *10 minutes*
Cooking time: *0 minutes*
Servings: *4*
Ingredients:

- 2 cups chives, chopped
- 1/2 cup almond milk

- ¼ cup chopped carrot
- ¼ cup chopped red onion
- Salt and black pepper to the taste
- 1 teaspoon sweet paprika

Directions:

1. In a blender, mix the chives with the carrot and the other ingredients and blend well.
2. Divide into bowls and serve.

Nutrition: calories 210, fat 3.4, carbs 6.4, protein 6

Stuffed Avocado

Preparation time: 10 minutes
Cooking time: 0 minutes
Servings: 2
Ingredients:

- 2 avocados, halved, pitted and flesh scooped out
- ¼ cup chives, chopped
- ½ cup carrot, grated
- ½ cup kale, chopped
- 1 teaspoon dried thyme
- A pinch of salt and black pepper
- ¼ teaspoon cayenne pepper
- 1 teaspoon paprika
- Salt and black pepper to the taste
- 2 tablespoons lemon juice

Directions:

1. In a bowl, mix the chives with carrots, avocado flesh, and the other

ingredients except for the avocado shells and stir well.

2. Stuff the avocado skins with this mix, arrange them on a platter, and serve as an appetizer.

Nutrition: calories 160, fat 10, carbs 4,2, protein 5.5

Radish Chips

Preparation time: 10 minutes

Cooking time: 20 minutes

Servings: 4

Ingredients:

- 2 teaspoons avocado oil
- 15 radishes, sliced
- A pinch of salt and black pepper
- 1 tablespoon chopped chives

Directions:

1. Arrange radish slices on a lined baking sheet, add the other ingredients, toss and place in the oven at 375 degrees F.
2. Bake for 10 minutes on each side, divide into bowls and serve cold.

Nutrition: calories 30, fat 1, fiber 2, carbs 7, protein 1

Avocado Cream

Preparation time: 10 minutes

Cooking time: 10 minutes

Servings: 4

Ingredients:

- 2 avocados, pitted, peeled, and chopped
- 1 cup almond milk
- 2 scallions, chopped
- Salt and black pepper to the taste
- 2 tablespoons coconut oil
- 1 tablespoon chives, chopped

Directions:

1. Heat up a pot with the coconut oil over medium heat.

2. Add scallions and avocado and cook for 2 minutes.

Nutrition: calories 162, fat 4.4, carbs 6, protein 6

Spicy kale chips

Prep time: 10 min

Cooking time: 30 min

Serving: 2

Ingredients:

- 1 large head of curly kale, wash, dry, and pulled from stem 1 tbsp extra virgin olive oil
- Minced parsley
- Squeeze of lemon juice
- Cayenne pepper
- Dash of soy sauce

Directions:

1. In a large bowl, rip the kale from the stem into palm-sized pieces.
2. Sprinkle the minced parsley, olive oil, soy sauce, a squeeze lemon juice, and a very small pinch of the cayenne powder.
3. Toss with a set of tongs or salad forks, and make sure to coat all of the leaves.
4. If you have a dehydrator, turn it on to 118F, spread out the kale on a dehydrator sheet, and leave it there for about 2 hours.
5. If you are cooking them, place parchment paper on top of a cookie sheet.
6. Lay the bed of kale and separate it a bit to make sure the kale is evenly toasted.
7. Cook for 10-15 minutes maximum at 250F.

Nutrition: Calories 284, Fat 5, Carbs 16, Protein 21

Sweet and Savory Guacamole

Preparation time: 10 minutes
Cooking time: 15 minutes
Serving: 2
Ingredients:

- 2 large avocados, pitted and scooped
- 2 Medjool dates, pitted and sliced into pieces
- ½ cup cherry tomatoes, cut into halves
- 5 sprigs of parsley, chopped
- ¼ cup of arugula, chopped
- 5 sticks of celery, washed, cut into sticks for dipping
- Juice from ¼ lime
- Dash of sea salt

Directions:

1. Mash the avocado in a bowl, sprinkle salt, and squeeze lime juice.
2. Fold in the tomatoes, dates, herbs, and greens.
3. Scoop with celery sticks, and enjoy!

Nutrition: Calories 233, Fat 2, Carbs 2, Protein 6

Mushroom Scramble Eggs

Preparation time: 5 minutes
Cooking time: 30 minutes
Serving: 2
Ingredients:

- 2 eggs
- 1 tsp ground turmeric
- 1 tsp mellow curry powder
- 20g kale, generally slashed
- 1 tsp additional virgin olive oil
- ½ superior bean stew, daintily cut
- A bunch of catch mushrooms, meagerly cut
- 5g parsley, finely slashed

Directions:

1. Blend the turmeric and curry powder and include a little water until you have accomplished a light glue.
2. Steam the kale for 2-3 minutes.
3. Warmth the oil in a skillet over medium heat and fry the bean stew and mushrooms for 2-3 minutes until they have begun to darker and mollify.
4. Include the eggs and flavor glue and cook over a medium warmth, at that point add the kale and keep on cooking over medium heat for a further moment. At long last, include the parsley, blend well and serve.

Nutrition: Calories 324, Fat 3, Carbs 10, Protein 23

Indian Lentil Soup

Preparation time: 10 min
Cooking time: 50 min
Servings: 2
Ingredients:

- 2 cups of lentils
- 1 small red onion, minced
- 1 stalk of celery, finely chopped
- 1 carrot, chopped
- 2 large leaves of kale, chopped finely
- 2 sprigs of cilantro, minced
- 3 sprigs of parsley, minced
- ¼-½ chili pepper, deseeded and minced
- 1 tomato, chopped into small pieces
- 1 chunk of ginger, minced
- 1 clove of garlic, minced
- 5 cups of chicken or vegetable stock
- 1 tsp of turmeric
- 1 tsp extra virgin olive oil
- ½ tsp Salt

Directions:

1. Cook lentils according to the package, remove from heat about 5 minutes before they would be done.
2. In a saucepan, sauté all of the vegetables in the olive oil.
3. Then add the chopped greens last.
4. Then add the ginger, garlic, and chill, and turmeric powder.
5. Add the stock and simmer for 5 minutes.
6. Add the lentils and salt.
7. Stir in the pre-cooked lentils and cook longer, on a very low simmer, for 25 more minutes.
8. Remove from the heat and cool.
9. Cut the avocado, remove the pit, and slice it, then scoop out the slices just before eating.
10. Top with avocado slice, then serve immediately.

Nutrition: Calories 234, Fat 2, Carbs 6, Protein 12

Buckwheat Noodles with Veggies

Preparation time: 20 min

Cooking time: 25 min

Servings: 2

Ingredients:

- 8 ounces buckwheat noodles
- 2 tablespoons olive oil
- 1 shallot, minced
- 1 cup fresh mushrooms, sliced
- 2 carrots, peeled and sliced diagonally
- 1½ cups bok choy, chopped
- 1/3 cup low-sodium vegetable broth
- 1 tablespoon low-sodium soy sauce

Directions:

1. Bring lightly salted water in a pan to boil, cook the soba noodles for about 5 minutes.
2. Drain the noodles well and rinse under cold water. Set aside.
3. Over medium heat, heat the oil in a large wok and sauté the shallots for about 3 minutes.
4. Add the mushrooms and stir-fry for about 4–5 minutes.
5. Add carrots and fry for 3 minutes while stirring.
6. Add bok choy and stir-fry for about 2–3 minutes.
7. Add broth and simmer for about 2 minutes. Add soy sauce and noodles and cook for about 1–2 minutes, tossing occasionally. Serve hot.

Nutrition: Calories 224, Fat 1, Carbs 2, Protein 6

Cheesy Mushrooms Caps

Preparation time: 10 min

Cooking time: 30 min

Servings: 2

Ingredients:

- 2 white mushroom caps
- 1 garlic clove, minced
- 3 tablespoons parsley, chopped
- 2 yellow onions, chopped
- Black pepper to the taste
- ½ cup low-fat parmesan, grated
- ¼ cup low-fat mozzarella, grated
- A drizzle of olive oil
- 2 tablespoons non-fat yogurt

Directions:

1. Heat up oil in a pan with over medium heat, add garlic and onion, stir, cook for 10 minutes and transfer to a bowl.
2. Add black pepper, garlic, parsley, mozzarella, parmesan, and yogurt, stir well, stuff the mushroom caps with this mix, arrange them on a lined baking sheet, bake in the oven at 400 degrees F for 20 minutes and serve.

Nutrition: Calories 220, Fat 3, Carbs 4, Protein 12

Beet Chips

Preparation time: *15 minutes*
Cooking time: *45 minutes*
Servings: 2
Ingredients:

- 2 big beets, peeled and thinly sliced
- Juice of 1 lemon
- 1 Serrano chili pepper, chopped
- ½ teaspoon fresh grated ginger
- A pinch of salt and black pepper
- 2 tablespoons avocado oil
- ¼ cup chopped cilantro

Directions:

1. Spread the chips on a lined baking sheet, toss and bake at 390 degrees F for 45 minutes.
2. Serve as a snack.

Nutrition: calories 160, fat 3, carbs 5, protein 5

Avocado and Radish Salsa

Preparation time: 10 minutes
Cooking time: 0 minutes
Servings: 4
Ingredients:

- 2 small avocados, pitted, peeled, and chopped
- 2 cups radishes, cubed
- 1 cup cucumber, cubed
- Juice of 1 lemon
- 1 tablespoon avocado oil
- 1 tablespoon chives, chopped
- 1 tablespoon cilantro, chopped

Directions:

1. In a bowl, mix the avocados with the radishes and the other ingredients, toss and serve.

Nutrition: calories 220, fat 6, carbs 12, protein 6

Tomato Platter

Preparation time: 10 minutes
Cooking time: 20 minutes
Servings: 6
Ingredients:

- 2 pounds cherry tomatoes, halved
- 1 teaspoon crushed red pepper flakes
- 3 garlic cloves, minced
- 1 handful chopped parsley
- 1 teaspoon curry powder
- 1 teaspoon sweet paprika
- Salt and black pepper to the taste
- 1 tablespoon avocado oil

Directions:

1. Spread the tomatoes on a lined baking sheet, add the rest of the ingredients, toss and roast at 400 degrees F for 20 minutes. Serve as an appetizer.

Nutrition: calories 170, fat 3.4, carbs 6, protein 5.5

Cauliflower and Broccoli Bites

Preparation time: *10 minutes*
Cooking time: *20 minutes*
Servings: *4*
Ingredients:

- 1 cup cauliflower florets
- 1 cup broccoli florets
- 2 tablespoons avocado oil
- 2 tablespoons green onions, chopped
- 1 teaspoon sweet paprika
- 1 tablespoon lemon juice
- A pinch of salt

Directions:

1. Spread the broccoli and cauliflower on a lined baking sheet, add the rest of the ingredients, toss and bake at 400 degrees F for 20 minutes.

2. Divide into bowls and serve as a snack.

Nutrition: calories 180, fat 6.6, carbs 6, protein 5.2

Chives Chutney

Preparation time: 10 minutes

Cooking time: 20 minutes

Servings: 10

Ingredients:

- 1 teaspoon cumin seeds
- 1 tablespoon avocado oil
- 1 cup chives, chopped
- ½ cup water
- 1 cup cherry tomatoes, cubed
- ½ teaspoon garam masala
- 1 teaspoon ground ginger
- ½ teaspoon cayenne pepper

Directions:

1. Heat up a pan with the oil over medium heat, add the chives and cumin, and cook for 5 minutes.
2. Add the rest of the ingredients, simmer the mixture over medium heat for 15 minutes more, divide into bowls, and serve cold.

Nutrition: calories 120, fat 4,4, carbs 5, protein 6

Blueberry Muffins

Preparation time: 35 minutes

Cooking time: 20 minutes

Servings: 12

Ingredients:

- 2 eggs
- 1/2 cup fresh blueberries
- 1 cup heavy cream
- 2 cups almond flour
- 1/4 tsp lemon zest
- 1/2 tsp lemon extract
- 1 tsp baking powder

- 5 drops stevia
- 1/4 cup butter, melted

Directions:

1. Preheat the oven to 350 F. Line muffin tin with cupcake liners and set aside.
2. Add eggs into the bowl and whisk until mix. Add remaining ingredients and mix to combine.
3. Pour mixture into the prepared muffin tin and bake for 25 minutes.
4. Serve and enjoy.

Nutrition: calories 190, Fat 17, Carbs 5, Protein 5

Chia Pudding

Preparation time: 15 minutes

Cooking time: 20 minutes

Servings: 2

Ingredients:

- 4 tbsp chia seeds
- 1 cup unsweetened coconut milk
- 1/2 cup raspberries

Directions:

1. Add raspberry and coconut milk into a blender and blend until smooth.
2. Pour mixture into the glass jar.
3. Add chia seeds in a jar and stir well.
4. Seal the jar with a lid and shake well and place in the refrigerator for 3 hours.
5. Serve chilled and enjoy.

Nutrition: calories 360, Fat 33, Carbs 13, Protein 6

Avocado Pudding

Preparation time: 10 minutes

Cooking time: 20 minutes

Servings: 10

Ingredients:

- 2 ripe avocados, peeled, pitted, and cut into pieces
- 1 tbsp fresh lime juice

- 14 oz can coconut milk
- 2 tsp liquid stevia
- 2 tsp vanilla

Directions:

1. Add all ingredients into the blender and blend until smooth.
2. Serve immediately and enjoy.

Nutrition: calories 317, Fat 30, Carbs 9, Protein 3

Peanut Butter Coconut Popsicle

Preparation time: 10 minutes
Cooking time: 20 minutes
Servings: 10
Ingredients:

- 1/2 cup peanut butter
- 1 tsp liquid stevia
- 2 cans unsweetened coconut milk

Directions:

1. Add all ingredients into the blender and blend until smooth.
2. Pour mixture into the Popsicle molds and place in the freezer for 4 hours or until set.
3. Serve and enjoy.

Nutrition: calories 155, Fat 15, Carbs 4, Protein 3

CHAPTER 4:

Optavia Lunch Recipes

Roasted Cornish Hen

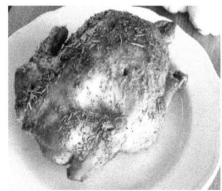

Preparation time: 15 minutes

Cooking time: 1 hour

Servings: 8

- 1 tablespoon dried basil, crushed
- 2 tablespoons lemon pepper
- 1 tablespoon poultry seasoning
- Salt, as required
- 4 (1½-pound) Cornish game hens, rinsed and dried completely
- 2 tablespoons olive oil
- 1 yellow onion, chopped
- 1 celery stalk, chopped
- 1 green bell pepper, seeded and chopped

Directions:

1. Preheat your oven to 375°F. Arrange lightly greased racks in 2 large roasting pans.
2. In a bowl, mix well basil, lemon pepper, poultry seasoning, and salt.
3. Coat each hen with oil and then rub evenly with the seasoning mixture.
4. In another bowl, mix together the onion, celery, and bell pepper.
5. Stuff the cavity of each hen loosely with veggie mixture.
6. Arrange the hens into prepared roasting pans, keeping plenty of space between them.
7. Roast for about 60 minutes or until the juices run clear.
8. Remove the hens from the oven and place them onto a cutting board.
9. With a foil piece, cover each hen loosely for about 10 minutes before carving.
10. Cut into desired size pieces and serve.

Nutrition: Calories 432, Fat 18, Carbs 4, Protein 23

Butter Chicken

Preparation time: 15 minutes

Cooking time: 28 minutes

Servings: 5

Ingredients:

- 3 tablespoons unsalted butter
- 1 medium yellow onion, chopped
- 2 garlic cloves, minced
- 1 teaspoon fresh ginger, minced
- 1½ pounds grass-fed chicken breasts, cut into ¾-inch chunks
- 2 tomatoes, chopped finely
- 1 tablespoon garam masala
- 1 teaspoon red chili powder
- 1 teaspoon ground cumin

- Salt and ground black pepper, as required
- 1 cup heavy cream
- 2 tablespoons fresh cilantro, chopped

Directions:

1. Melt butter in a large wok over medium-high heat and sauté the onions for about 5–6 minutes.
2. Now, add in ginger and garlic and sauté for about 1 minute.
3. Add the tomatoes and cook for about 2–3 minutes, crushing with the back of the spoon.
4. Stir in the chicken spices, salt, and black pepper, and cook for about 6–8 minutes or until the desired doneness of the chicken.
5. Stir in the heavy cream and cook for about 8–10 more minutes, stirring occasionally.
6. Garnish with fresh cilantro and serve hot.

Nutrition: Calories 506, Fat 22, Carbs 4, Protein 32

Turkey Chili

Preparation Time: 15 Minutes
Cooking Time: 120 Minutes
Servings: 8
Ingredients:

- 2 tablespoons olive oil
- 1 small yellow onion, chopped
- 1 green bell pepper, seeded and chopped
- 4 garlic cloves, minced
- 1 jalapeño pepper, chopped
- 1 teaspoon dried thyme, crushed
- 2 tablespoons red chili powder
- 1 tablespoon ground cumin
- 2 pounds lean ground turkey
- 2 cups fresh tomatoes, chopped finely

- 2 ounces' sugar-free tomato paste
- 2 cups homemade chicken broth
- 1 cup of water
- Salt and ground black pepper, as required
- 1 cup cheddar cheese, shredded

Directions:

1. In a large Dutch oven, heat oil over medium heat and sauté the onion and bell pepper for about 5–7 minutes.
2. Add the garlic, jalapeño pepper, thyme, and spices and sauté for about 1 minute.
3. Add the turkey and cook for about 4–5 minutes.
4. Stir in the tomatoes, tomato paste, and cacao powder, and cook for about 2 minutes.
5. Add in the broth and water and bring to a boil.
6. Now, reduce the heat to low and simmer, covered for about 2 hours.
7. Add in salt and black pepper and remove from the heat.
8. Top with cheddar cheese and serve hot.

Nutrition: Calories 308, Fat 20, Carbs 10, Protein 8

Beef Curry

Preparation time: 15 minutes
Cooking time: 2¼ hours
Servings: 8
Ingredients

- 2 tablespoons olive oil
- 1 small yellow onion, chopped
- 1 green bell pepper, seeded and chopped
- 4 garlic cloves, minced
- 1 jalapeño pepper, chopped
- 1 teaspoon dried thyme, crushed
- 2 tablespoons red chili powder
- 1 tablespoon ground cumin

- 2 pounds lean ground turkey
- 2 cups fresh tomatoes, chopped finely
- 2 ounces sugar-free tomato paste
- 2 cups homemade chicken broth
- 1 cup water
- Salt and ground black pepper, as required
- 1 cup cheddar cheese, shredded

Directions:

1. In a large Dutch oven, heat oil over medium heat and sauté the onion and bell pepper for about 5–7 minutes.
2. Add the garlic, jalapeño pepper, thyme, and spices and sauté for about 1 minute.
3. Add the turkey and cook for about 4–5 minutes.
4. Stir in the tomatoes, tomato paste, and cacao powder, and cook for about 2 minutes.
5. Add in the broth and water and bring to a boil.
6. Now, reduce the heat to low and simmer, covered for about 2 hours.
7. Add in salt and black pepper and remove from the heat.
8. Top with cheddar cheese and serve hot.

Nutrition: Calories 234, Fat 12, Carbs 4, Protein 24

Shepherd's pie

Preparation time: 20 minutes
Cooking time: 50 minutes
Servings: 6
Ingredients:

- ¼ cup olive oil
- 1 pound grass-fed ground beef
- ½ cup celery, chopped
- ¼ cup yellow onion, chopped
- 3 garlic cloves, minced
- 1 cup tomatoes, chopped

- 2 (12-ounce) packages riced cauliflower, cooked and well drained
- 1 cup cheddar cheese, shredded
- ¼ cup Parmesan cheese, shredded
- 1 cup heavy cream
- 1 teaspoon dried thyme

Directions:

1. Preheat your oven to 350°F.
2. Heat oil in a large nonstick wok over medium heat and cook the ground beef, celery, onions, and garlic for about 8–10 minutes.
3. Remove from the heat and drain the excess grease.
4. Immediately stir in the tomatoes.
5. Transfer mixture into a 10x7-inch casserole dish evenly.
6. In a food processor, add the cauliflower, cheeses, cream, and thyme, and pulse until a mashed potatoes-like mixture is formed.
7. Spread the cauliflower mixture over the meat in the casserole dish evenly.
8. Bake for about 35–40 minutes.
9. Remove casserole dish from oven and let it cool slightly before serving.
10. Cut into desired sized pieces and serve.

Nutrition: Calories 404, Fat 5, Carbs 9, Protein 23

Meatballs Curry

Preparation time: 15 minutes
Cooking time: 25 minutes
Servings: 6
Meatballs

- 1 pound lean ground pork
- 2 organic eggs, beaten
- 3 tablespoons yellow onion, finely chopped
- ¼ cup fresh parsley leaves, chopped
- ¼ teaspoon fresh ginger, minced

- 2 garlic cloves, minced
- 1 jalapeño pepper, seeded and finely chopped
- 1 teaspoon granulated erythritol
- 1 teaspoon curry powder
- 3 tablespoons olive oil

Curry

- 1 yellow onion, chopped
- Salt, as required
- 2 garlic cloves, minced
- ¼ teaspoon fresh ginger, minced
- 1 tablespoon curry powder
- 1 (14-ounce) can unsweetened coconut milk
- Ground black pepper, as required
- ¼ cup fresh parsley, minced

Directions:

For meatballs:

1. Place all the ingredients (except oil) in a large bowl and mix until well combined.
2. Make small-sized balls from the mixture.
3. Heat the oil in a large wok over medium heat and cook meatballs for about 3–5 minutes or until golden-brown from all sides.
4. Transfer the meatballs into a bowl.

For curry:

5. In the same wok, add onion and a pinch of salt, and sauté for about 4–5 minutes.
6. Add the garlic and ginger, and sauté for about 1 minute.
7. Add the curry powder and sauté for about 1–2 minutes.
8. Add coconut milk and meatballs, and bring to a gentle simmer.
9. Adjust the heat to low and simmer, covered for about 10–12 minutes.

10. Season with salt and black pepper and remove from the heat.
11. Top with parsley and serve.

Nutrition: Calories 350, Fat 13, Carbs 6, Protein 16

Pork with Veggies

Preparation time: 15 minutes
Cooking time: 15 minutes
Servings: 5
Ingredients

- 1 pound pork loin, cut into thin strips
- 2 tablespoons olive oil, divided
- 1 teaspoon garlic, minced
- 1 teaspoon fresh ginger, minced
- 2 tablespoons low-sodium soy sauce
- 1 tablespoon fresh lemon juice
- 1 teaspoon sesame oil
- 1 tablespoon granulated erythritol
- 1 teaspoon arrowroot starch
- 10 ounces broccoli florets
- 1 carrot, peeled and sliced
- 1 large red bell pepper, seeded and cut into strips
- 2 scallions, cut into 2-inch pieces

Directions:

1. In a bowl, mix well pork strips, ½ tablespoon of olive oil, garlic, and ginger.
2. For sauce: Add the soy sauce, lemon juice, sesame oil, Swerve, and arrowroot starch in a small bowl and mix well.
3. Heat the remaining olive oil in a large nonstick wok over high heat and sear the pork strips for about 3–4 minutes or until cooked through.
4. With a slotted spoon, transfer the pork into a bowl.
5. In the same wok, add the carrot and cook for about 2–3 minutes.

6. Add the broccoli, bell pepper, and scallion, and cook, covered for about 1–2 minutes.

7. Stir the cooked pork, sauce, and stir-fry, and cook for about 3–5 minutes or until the desired doneness, stirring occasionally.

8. Remove from the heat and serve.

Nutrition: Calories 315, Fat 19, Carbs 11, Protein 27

Pork Taco Bake

Preparation time: 15 minutes

Cooking time: 1 hour

Servings: 6

Ingredients

- 3 organic eggs
- ½ teaspoon taco seasoning
- 4 ounces canned chopped green chilies
- ¼ cup sugar-free tomato sauce
- 3 teaspoons taco seasoning
- 8 ounces cheddar cheese, shredded
- ¼ cup fresh basil leaves

Directions:

1. Preheat your oven to 375°F.
2. Lightly grease a 13x9-inch baking dish.
3. For crust: In a bowl, add the eggs and cream cheese, and beat until well combined and smooth.
4. Add the taco seasoning and heavy cream, and mix well.
5. Place cheddar cheese evenly in the bottom of the prepared baking dish.
6. Spread cream cheese mixture evenly over cheese.
7. Bake for about 25–30 minutes.
8. Remove baking dish from the oven and set aside for about 5 minutes.
9. Meanwhile, for the topping: Heat a large nonstick wok over medium-high heat and cook the pork for about 8–10 minutes.

10. Drain the excess grease from the wok.
11. Stir in the green chilies, tomato sauce, and taco seasoning, and remove from the heat.
12. Place the pork mixture evenly over the crust and sprinkle with cheese.
13. Bake for about 18–20 minutes or until bubbly.
14. Remove from the oven and set aside for about 5 minutes.
15. Cut into desired size slices and serve with the garnishing of basil leaves.

Nutrition: Calories 556, Fat 39, Carbs 5, Protein 43

Spinach Pie

Preparation time: 15 minutes

Cooking time: 38 minutes

Servings: 5

Ingredients:

- 2 tablespoons butter, divided
- 2 tablespoons yellow onion, chopped
- 1 (16-ounce) bag frozen chopped spinach, thawed and squeezed
- 1½ cups heavy cream
- 3 organic eggs
- ½ teaspoon ground nutmeg
- Salt and ground black pepper, as required
- ½ cup Swiss cheese, shredded

Directions:

1. Preheat your oven to 375°F.
2. Grease a 9-inch baking dish.
3. In a large wok, melt 1 tablespoon of butter over medium-high heat and sauté onion for about 4–5 minutes.
4. Add spinach and cook for about 2–3 minutes or until all the liquid is absorbed.
5. In a bowl, add cream, eggs, nutmeg, salt, and black pepper, and beat until well combined.

6. Transfer the spinach mixture to the bottom of the prepared baking dish evenly.
7. Place the egg mixture over the spinach mixture evenly and sprinkle with cheese.
8. Top with remaining butter in the shape of dots at many places.
9. Bake for about 25–30 minutes or until the top becomes golden brown.

Nutrition: Calories 267, Fat 9, Carbs 1, Protein 24

Baked Chicken Fajitas

Preparation time: 10 minutes
Cooking time: 18 minutes
Servings: 6
Ingredients:

- 1 1/2 lbs chicken tenders
- 2 tbsp fajita seasoning
- 2 tbsp olive oil
- 1 onion, sliced
- 2 bell pepper, sliced
- 1 lime juice
- 1 tsp kosher salt

Directions:

1. Preheat the oven to 400 F.
2. Add all ingredients in a large mixing bowl and toss well.
3. Transfer bowl mixture on a baking tray and bake in preheated oven for 15-18 minutes. Serve and enjoy.

Nutrition: Calories 286, Fat 13, Carbs 7, Protein 33

Pesto Zucchini Noodles

Preparation Time: 5 Minutes
Cooking Time: 2 Minutes
Servings: 4
Ingredients:

- 3 lbs Zucchini

- Spiral Slicer
- Olive Oil

Directions:

1. Prepare the Zucchini: trim the ends away from your zucchini.
2. Using the instructions to your spiral slicer, slice the zucchini into noodles. Store, Or Cook: Simply heat a saucepan with olive oil over medium heat. Saute zoodles for 5 minutes, until tender!

Nutrition: Calories 56, Fat 1, Carbs 11, Protein 2

Sautéd Crispy Zucchini

Preparation time: 15 minutes
Cooking time: 38 minutes
Servings: 5
Ingredients:

- 2 tbsp. butter
- 4 zucchini, cut into 1/4-in.-thick rounds
- 1/4 c. freshly grated Parmesan cheese
- Freshly ground black pepper

Directions

1. In a large skillet over medium-high heat, melt butter.
2. Add zucchini and cook, stirring occasionally, until tender and lightly browned, about 5 min.
3. Spread zucchini evenly in skillet and sprinkle Parmesan over vegetables.
4. Cook without stirring until Parmesan is melted and crispy where it touches skillet, about 5 min. Top with pepper and serve.

Nutrition: Calories 156, Fat 4, Carbs 0, Protein 2

Easy Low Carb Cauliflower Pizza Crust

Preparation time: 15 minutes

Cooking time: 8 minutes

Servings: 8

Ingredients:

- 3 cups almond flour
- 3 tbsp butter, then melted
- ⅓ tsp salt
- Cauliflower
- 3 large eggs

Directions

1. Preheat oven to 350°F. In a bowl, mix the almond flour, butter, salt, and eggs until a dough forms. Mold the dough into a ball and place it in between two wide parchment papers on a flat surface. Place the cauliflower on the dough.
2. Use a rolling pin to roll it out into a circle of a quarter-inch thickness. Place the cauliflower on the dough.
3. Slide the pizza dough into the pizza pan and remove the parchment papers. Bake the dough for 20 minutes.

Nutrition: Calories 234, Fat 16, Carbs 8, Protein 12

Fresh Tomato Basil Soup

Preparation time: 15 minutes

Cooking time: 40 minutes

Servings: 4

Ingredients:

- ¼ c. olive oil
- ½ c. heavy cream
- 1 lb. tomatoes, fresh
- 4 c. chicken broth, divided
- 4 cloves garlic, fresh
- Sea salt & pepper to taste

Directions:

1. Preheat oven to 400° Fahrenheit and line a baking sheet with foil.
2. Remove the cores from your tomatoes and place them on the baking sheet along with the cloves of garlic.
3. Drizzle tomatoes and garlic with olive oil, salt, and pepper.
4. Roast for 30 minutes.
5. Pull the tomatoes out of the oven and place them into a blender, along with the juices that have dripped onto the pan during roasting.
6. Add two cups of the chicken broth to the blender.
7. Blend until smooth, then strain the mixture into a large saucepan or a pot.
8. While the pan is on the stove, whisk the remaining two cups of broth and the cream into the soup.
9. Simmer for about ten minutes.
10. Season to taste, then serve hot!

Nutrition: Calories 255, Fat 20, Carbs 6, Protein 7

Creamy Beef Stroganoff

Preparation time: 10 minutes

Cooking time: 20 minutes

Servings: 4

Ingredients:

- 1 lb beef strips
- 3/4 cup mushrooms, sliced
- 1 small onion, chopped
- 1 tbsp butter
- 2 tbsp olive oil
- 2 tbsp green onion, chopped
- 1/4 cup sour cream
- 1 cup chicken broth
- Pepper
- Salt

Directions:

1. Add meat in bowl and coat with 1 teaspoon oil, pepper, and salt.
2. Heat remaining oil in a pan.
3. Add meat to the pan and cook until golden brown on both sides.
4. Transfer meat to a bowl and set aside.
5. Add butter to the same pan.
6. Add onion and cook until onion softened.
7. Add mushrooms and sauté until the liquid is absorbed.
8. Add broth and cook until the sauce thickened.
9. Add sour cream, green onion, and meat and stir well.
10. Cook over medium-high heat for 3-4 minutes.
11. Serve and enjoy.

Nutrition: Calories 345, Fat 20, Carbs 3, Protein 35

Quick Veggie Protein Bowl

Preparation time: 5 minutes
Cooking time: 13 minutes
Servings: 1
Ingredients:

- 4 oz. extra-firm tofu, drained
- ¼ tsp. turmeric
- ¼ tsp. cayenne pepper
- 1 tbsp. coconut oil
- 1 cup broccoli florets, diced
- 1 cup Chinese kale, diced
- ½ cup button mushrooms, diced
- ½ tsp. dried oregano
- Himalayan salt
- Black pepper to taste
- ½ tsp. paprika
- ¼ cup of fresh oregano, diced

Directions:

1. Cut the tofu into tiny pieces and season with turmeric and cayenne pepper.
2. Warm a large skillet and add ¾ of the coconut oil.
3. Once the oil is heated, add the tofu and cook it for about 5 minutes, stirring continuously.
4. Transfer the cooked tofu to a medium-sized bowl and set it aside.
5. Add the remaining coconut oil, diced broccoli florets, Chinese kale, button mushrooms, and the remaining herbs to the skillet. Use paprika, pepper, and salt to taste.
6. Cook the vegetables for 6-8 minutes, stirring continuously.
7. Transfer the cooked veggies and tofu to the bowl. Garnish with the optional fresh oregano.
8. Serve and enjoy!

Nutrition: Calories 596, Fat 20, Carbs 6, Protein 17

Pork Bowls

Preparation time: 15 minutes
Cooking time: 15 minutes
Servings: 4
Ingredients:

- 1¼ pounds pork belly, cut into bite-size pieces
- 2 Tbsp tamari soy sauce
- 1 Tbsp rice vinegar
- 2 cloves garlic, smashed
- 3 oz butter
- 1 pound Brussels sprouts, rinsed, trimmed, halved, or quartered
- ½ leek, chopped
- Salt and ground black pepper to taste

Directions:

1. Fry the pork over medium-high heat until it is starting to turn golden brown.

2. Combine the garlic cloves, butter, and brussel sprouts. Add to the pan, whisk well and cook until the sprouts turn golden brown.

3. Stir the soy sauce and rice vinegar together and pour the sauce into the pan.

4. Sprinkle with salt and pepper. Top with chopped leek.

Nutrition: Calories 421, Fat 22, Carbs 7, Protein 19

CHAPTER 5:

Optavia Dinner Recipes

Mussels in Red Wine Sauce

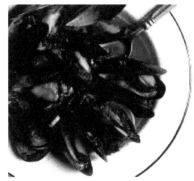

Preparation time: 5 minutes
Cooking time: 5 minutes
Servings: 2
Ingredients:

- 800g mussels
- 2 x 400g tins of chopped tomatoes
- 25g butter
- 1 fresh chives, chopped
- 1 fresh parsley, chopped
- 1 bird's-eye chili, finely chopped
- 4 cloves of garlic, crushed
- 400mls red wine
- Juice of 1 lemon

Directions:

1. Wash the mussels, remove their beards, and set them aside. Heat the butter in a large saucepan and add in the red wine. Reduce the heat and add the parsley, chives, chili, and garlic whilst stirring. Add in the tomatoes, lemon juice, and mussels. Cover the saucepan and cook for 2-3. Remove the saucepan from the heat and take out any mussels which haven't opened and discard them. Serve and eat immediately.

Nutrition: calories: 364, carbs: 3.3, Fat: 4.9, Protein: 8

Roast Balsamic Vegetables
Preparation time: 10 minutes
Cooking time: 45 minutes
Servings: 4
Ingredients:

- 4 tomatoes, chopped 2 red onions, chopped
- 3 sweet potatoes, peeled and chopped
- 100g red chicory (or if unavailable, use yellow)
- 100g kale, finely chopped
- 300g potatoes, peeled and chopped
- 5 stalks of celery, chopped
- 1 bird's-eye chili, de-seeded and finely chopped
- 2g fresh parsley, chopped
- 2gs fresh coriander (cilantro) chopped
- 3 teaspoons olive oil
- 2 teaspoons balsamic vinegar
- 1 teaspoon mustard Sea salt
- Freshly ground black pepper

Directions:

1. Place the olive oil, balsamic, mustard, parsley, and coriander (cilantro) into a bowl and mix well. Toss all the

remaining ingredients into the dressing and season with salt and pepper. Transfer the vegetables to an ovenproof dish and cook in the oven at 200C/400F for 45 minutes.

Nutrition: Calories: 310, carbs: 1, Protein: 0.2g

Tomato and Goat's Pizza

Preparation time: 15 minutes
Cooking time: 20 minutes
Servings: 2
Ingredients:

- 225g buckwheat flour
- 2 teaspoons dried yeast Pinch of salt
- 150mls slightly water 1 teaspoon olive oil

For the Topping:

- 75g feta cheese, crumbled
- 75g peseta (or tomato paste)
- 1 tomato, sliced 1 red onion, finely chopped
- 25g rocket (arugula) leaves, chopped

Directions:

1. In a bowl, combine all the ingredients for the pizza dough, then allow it to stand for at least an hour until it has doubled in size. Roll the dough out to a size to suit you. Spoon the passata onto the base and add the rest of the toppings. Bake in the oven at 200C/400F for 15-20 minutes or until browned at the edges and crispy and serve.

Nutrition: Calories: 585 carbs: 77 Fat: 8, Protein: 22.9

Tender Spiced Lamb

Preparation time: 20 minutes
Cooking time: 4 hours 20 minutes
Servings: 8
Ingredients:

- 1.35kg lamb shoulder
- 3 red onions, sliced
- 3 cloves of garlic, crushed
- 1 bird's eye chili, finely chopped
- 1 teaspoon turmeric
- 1 teaspoon ground cumin
- ½ teaspoon ground coriander (cilantro)
- ¼ teaspoon ground cinnamon

Directions:

1. In a bowl, combine the chili, garlic, and spices with olive oil. Coat the lamb with the spice mixture and marinate it for an hour, or overnight if you can. Heat the remaining oil in a pan, add the lamb and brown it for 3-4 minutes on all sides to seal it. Place the lamb in an ovenproof dish. Add in the red onions and cover the dish with foil. Transfer to the oven and roast at 170C/325F for 4 hours. The lamb should be extremely tender and falling off the bone. Serve with rice or couscous, salad or vegetables.

Nutrition: calories: 455, carbs 28, Fat: 9.8 Protein: 20

Chili Cod Fillets

Preparation time: 10 minutes
Cooking time: 10 minutes
Servings: 4
Ingredients:

- 4 cod fillets
- 2 teaspoons fresh parsley, chopped
- 2 bird's-eye chilies (or more if you like it hot)
- 2 cloves of garlic, chopped
- 4 teaspoons olive oil

Directions:

1. Heat olive oil in a frying pan, add the fish, and cook for 7-8 minutes or until thoroughly cooked, turning once halfway through. Remove and keep

warm. Pour the remaining olive oil into the pan and add the chili, chopped garlic, and parsley. Warm it thoroughly. Serve the fish onto plates and pour the warm chili oil over it.

Nutrition: calories: 246, carbs: 5, Fat: 0.5, Protein: 18

Steak and Mushroom Noodles

Preparation time: 10 minutes

Cooking time: 20 minutes

Servings: 4

Ingredients:

- 100g shitake mushrooms, halved, if large
- 100g chestnut mushrooms, sliced
- 150g udon noodles
- 75g kale, finely chopped
- 75g baby leaf spinach, chopped
- 2 sirloin steaks
- 2 teaspoons miso paste
- 2.5cm piece fresh ginger, finely chopped
- 1 star anise
- 1 red chili, finely sliced
- 1 red onion, finely chopped
- 1 fresh coriander (cilantro) chopped
- 1 liter (1½ pints) warm water

Directions:

1. Pour the water into a saucepan and add in the miso, star anise, and ginger. Bring it to the boil, reduce the heat, and simmer gently. In the meantime, cook the noodles according to their instructions, then drain them.
2. Heat the oil in a saucepan, add the steak and cook for around 2-3 minutes on each side (or 1-2 minutes, for rare meat).
3. Remove the meat and set aside.

4. Place the mushrooms, spinach, coriander (cilantro), and kale into the miso broth and cook for 5 minutes.
5. In the meantime, heat the remaining oil in a separate pan and fry the chili and onion for 4 minutes, until softened.
6. Serve the noodles into bowls and pour the soup on top.
7. Thinly slice the steaks and add them to the top. Serve immediately.

Nutrition: calories: 296, carbs: 24, Fat: 13, Protein: 32

Masala Scallops

Preparation time: 10 minutes

Cooking time: 20 minutes

Servings: 4

Ingredients:

- 2 jalapenos, chopped
- 1 pound sea scallops
- A pinch of salt and black pepper
- ¼ teaspoon cinnamon powder
- 1 teaspoon garam masala
- 1 teaspoon coriander, ground
- 1 teaspoon cumin, ground
- 2 tablespoons cilantro, chopped

Directions:

1. Heat up a pan with the oil over medium heat, add the jalapenos, cinnamon, and the other ingredients except for the scallops and cook for 10 minutes.

Nutrition: Calories: 251, Fat: 4g, Carbs: 11g, Protein: 17g

Tuna and Tomatoes

Preparation time: 5 minutes

Cooking time: 20 minutes

Servings: 4

Ingredients:

- 1 yellow onion, chopped
- 1 tablespoon olive oil

- 1 cup tomatoes, chopped
- 1 red pepper, chopped
- 1 teaspoon sweet paprika
- 1 tablespoon coriander, chopped

Directions:
1. Heat up a pan with the oil over medium heat, add the onions and the pepper and cook for 5 minutes.
2. Add the fish and the other ingredients, cook everything for 15 minutes, divide between plates and serve.

Nutrition: Calories: 215, Fat: 4g, Carbs: 14g, Protein: 7g

Lemongrass and Ginger Mackerel
Preparation time: 10 minutes
Cooking time: 25 minutes
Servings: 4
Ingredients:
- 4 mackerel fillets, skinless and boneless
- 1 tablespoon ginger, grated
- 2 lemongrass sticks, chopped
- 2 red chilies, chopped
- Juice of 1 lime
- A handful parsley, chopped

Directions:
1. In a roasting pan, combine the mackerel with the oil, ginger, and the other ingredients, toss and bake at 390 degrees F for 25 minutes. Divide everything between plates and serve.

Nutrition: Calories: 251, Fat: 3, Carbs: 14, Protein: 8

Scallops with Almonds and Mushrooms
Preparation time: 5 minutes
Cooking time: 10 minutes
Servings: 4
Ingredients:
- 1 pound scallops

- 4 scallions, chopped
- A pinch of salt and black pepper
- ½ cup mushrooms, sliced
- 2 tablespoon almonds, chopped
- 1 cup coconut cream

Directions:
1. Heat up a pan with the oil over medium heat, add the scallions and the mushrooms and sauté for 2 minutes.

Nutrition: Calories: 322, Fat: 23.7, Carbs: 8.1, Protein: 21.6

Scallops and Sweet Potatoes
Preparation time: 5 minutes
Cooking time: 22 minutes
Servings: 4
Ingredients:
- 1 pound scallops
- 2 tablespoons avocado oil
- 1 yellow onion, chopped
- 2 sweet potatoes, peeled and cubed
- ½ cup chicken stock
- 1 tablespoon cilantro, chopped

Directions:
1. Heat up a pan with the oil over medium heat, add the onion and sauté for 2 minutes.
2. Add the sweet potatoes and the stock, toss and cook for 10 minutes more.

Nutrition: Calories: 211, Fat 4, Carbs: 26, Protein: 20

Salmon and Shrimp Salad
Preparation time: 5 minutes
Cooking time: 0 minutes
Servings: 4
Ingredients:
- 1 cup smoked salmon, boneless and flaked

- 1 cup shrimp, peeled, deveined and cooked
- ½ cup baby arugula
- 1 tablespoon lemon juice
- 2 spring onions, chopped
- 1 tablespoon olive oil
- A pinch of sea salt and black pepper

Directions:

1. In a salad bowl, combine the salmon with the shrimp and the other ingredients, toss and serve.

Nutrition: Calories: 210, Fat: 6, Carbs: 10, Protein: 1

Shrimp, Tomato and Dates Salad

Preparation time: 10 minutes

Cooking time: 0 minutes

Servings: 4

Ingredients:

- 1 pound shrimp, cooked, peeled, and deveined
- 2 cups baby spinach
- 2 tablespoons walnuts, chopped
- 1 cup cherry tomatoes, halved
- 1 tablespoon lemon juice
- ½ cup dates, chopped
- 2 tablespoons avocado oil

Directions:

1. In a salad bowl, mix the shrimp with the spinach, walnuts, and the other ingredients, toss and serve.

Nutrition: Calories: 243, Fat: 5.4g, Carbs: 21.6g, Protein: 28.3g

Salmon and Watercress Salad

Preparation time: 15 minutes

Cooking time: 0 minutes

Servings: 2

Ingredients: 2 spring onions, chopped

- 1 cup watercress

- 1 tablespoon lemon juice
- 1 cucumber, sliced
- 1 avocado, peeled, pitted and roughly cubed
- A pinch of sea salt and black pepper

Directions:

1. In a salad bowl, mix the salmon with the spring onions, watercress, and the other ingredients, toss and serve.

Nutrition: Calories: 261, Fat: 15, Carbs: 8, Protein: 22

Green Onion Soup

Preparation time: 5 minutes

Cooking time: 12 minutes

Servings: 2

Ingredients:

- 6 green onions, chopped
- 7 ounces diced potatoes
- 1/3 teaspoon salt
- 2 tablespoons olive oil
- 1 ¼ cup vegetable broth
- ¼ teaspoon ground white pepper
- ¼ teaspoon ground coriander

Directions

1. Take a small pan, place potato in it, cover with water, and then place the pan over medium heat.
2. Boil the potato until cooked and tender, and when done, drain the potatoes and set aside until required.
3. Return saucepan over low heat, add oil, and when hot, add green onions and cook for 5 minutes until cooked.
4. Season with salt, pepper, and coriander, add potatoes, pour in vegetable broth, stir until mixed and bring it to simmer.
5. Taste to adjust seasoning, then ladle soup into bowls and then serve

Nutrition: calories 191, fat 2, carbs 2, protein 15

Mashed Potatoes

Preparation time: 10 minutes
Cooking time: 12 minutes
Servings: 2
Ingredients:

- 4 potatoes, halved
- ¼ tablespoons chives, chopped
- 1 teaspoon minced garlic
- ¾ teaspoon sea salt
- 2 tablespoons butter, unsalted
- ¼ teaspoon ground black pepper

Directions:

1. Take a medium pot, place it over medium-high heat, add potatoes, cover with water and boil until cooked and tender.
2. When done, drain the potatoes, let them cool for 10 minutes, peel them and return them to the pot.
3. Mash the potatoes by using a hand mixer until fluffy, add remaining ingredients except for chives, and then stir until mixed.
4. Sprinkle chives over the top and then serve.

Nutrition: calories 396, fat 5, carbs 10, protein 23

Eggplant Stacks

Preparation time: 5 minutes
Cooking time: 10 minutes
Servings: 2
Ingredients:

- ½ pound, eggplant
- ½ teaspoon dried thyme
- ½ teaspoon dried oregano
- 2 tablespoons olive oil
- 4 tablespoons grated parmesan cheese
- ½ teaspoon salt
- ½ teaspoon ground black pepper

Directions:

1. Cut eggplant into 1-inch thick slices, brush them with oil and then sprinkle with salt, black pepper, thyme, and oregano on both until well-seasoned.
2. Then top eggplant slices with cheese, cover with a lid, and grill for 1 to 2 minutes until cheese has melted.

Nutrition: calories 200, fat 4, carbs 3, protein 7

Potato Soup

Preparation time: 5 minutes
Cooking time: 12 minutes
Servings: 2
Ingredients:

- 2 potatoes, peeled, cubed
- 1/3 teaspoon salt
- 4 teaspoons grated parmesan cheese
- 1 ½ cup vegetable broth
- ¾ cup of water
- 1/8 teaspoon ground black pepper
- 1 tablespoon Cajun seasoning

Directions

1. Take a small pan, place potato cubes in it, cover with water and vegetable broth, and then place the pan over medium heat. Return pan over medium-low heat, add remaining ingredients, stir until mixed and bring it to a simmer.
2. Taste to adjust seasoning, then ladle soup into bowls and then serve.

Nutrition: calories 210, fat 7, carbs 5, protein 18

Teriyaki Eggplant

Preparation time: 5 minutes
Cooking time: 15 minutes
Servings: 2
Ingredients:

- ½ pound eggplant

- 1 green onion, chopped
- ½ teaspoon grated ginger
- ½ teaspoon minced garlic
- 1/3 cup soy sauce
- 1 tablespoon coconut sugar
- ½ tablespoon apple cider vinegar
- 1 tablespoon olive oil

Directions:

1. Prepare teriyaki sauce and for this, take a medium bowl, add ginger, garlic, soy sauce, vinegar, and sugar in it and then whisk until sugar has dissolved completely.
2. Cut eggplant into cubes, add them into teriyaki sauce, toss until well coated, and marinate for 10 minutes.
3. When ready to cook, take a grill pan, place it over medium-high heat, grease it with oil, and when hot, add marinated eggplant. Cook for 3 to 4 minutes per side until nicely browned and beginning to charred, drizzling with excess marinade frequently and transfer to a plate.
4. Sprinkle green onion on top of the eggplant and then serve.

Nutrition: calories 126, fat 4, carbs 4, protein 13

Dijon Mustard and Lime Marinated Shrimp

Preparation Time: 10 minutes

Cooking Time: 10 minutes

Servings: 8

Ingredients:

- ½ cup fresh lime juice, and lime zest as garnish
- ½ cup rice vinegar
- ½ teaspoon hot sauce
- 1 bay leaf
- 1 cup water

- 1 lb. uncooked shrimp, peeled and deveined
- 1 medium red onion, chopped
- 2 tablespoon capers
- 2 tablespoon Dijon mustard
- 3 whole cloves

Directions:

1. Mix hot sauce, mustard, capers, lime juice and onion in a shallow baking dish and set aside.
2. Bring to a boil in a large saucepan bay leaf, cloves, vinegar and water.
3. Once boiling, add shrimps and cook for a minute while stirring continuously.
4. Drain shrimps and pour shrimps into onion mixture.
5. For an hour, refrigerate while covered the shrimps.
6. Then serve shrimps cold and garnished with lime zest.

Nutrition: Calories: 232.2 Protein: 17.8g Fat: 3g Carbs: 15g

Dill Relish on White Sea Bass

Preparation Time: 10 minutes

Cooking Time: 12 minutes

Servings: 4

Ingredients:

1 ½ tablespoon chopped white onion

1 ½ teaspoon chopped fresh dill

1 lemon, quartered

1 teaspoon Dijon mustard

1 teaspoon lemon juice

1 teaspoon pickled baby capers, drained

4 pieces of 4-oz white sea bass fillets

Directions:

Preheat oven to 375oF.

Mix lemon juice, mustard, dill, capers and onions in a small bowl.

Prepare four aluminum foil squares and place 1 fillet per foil.

Squeeze a lemon wedge per fish.

Evenly divide into 4 the dill spread and drizzle over fillet.

Close the foil over the fish securely and pop in the oven.

Bake for 12 minutes or until fish is cooked through.

Remove from foil and transfer to a serving platter, serve and enjoy.

Nutrition:

Calories: 115

Protein: 7g

Fat: 1g

Carbs: 12g

Quinoa With Vegetables

Preparation Time: 10 minutes

Cooking Time: 5 to 6 hours

Servings: 8

Ingredients:

2 cups quinoa, rinsed and drained

2 onions, chopped

2 carrots, peeled and sliced

1 cup sliced cremini mushrooms

3 garlic cloves, minced

4 cups low-sodium vegetable broth

1/2 teaspoon salt

1 teaspoon dried marjoram leaves

1/8 teaspoon freshly ground black pepper

Directions:

In a 6-quart slow cooker, mix all of the ingredients.

Cover and cook on low for 5 to 6 hours, or until the quinoa and vegetables are tender.

Stir the mixture and serve.

Nutrition:

Calories: 204 Cal

Carbohydrates: 35 g

Sugar: 4 g Fiber: 4 g

Fat: 3 g Saturated Fat: 0 g

Protein: 7 g Sodium: 229 mg

Chicken Goulash

Preparation Time: 10 minutes

Cooking Time: 17 minutes

Servings: 6

Ingredients:

4 oz. chive stems

2 green peppers, chopped

1 teaspoon olive oil

14 oz. ground chicken

2 tomatoes

½ cup chicken stock

2 garlic cloves, sliced

1 teaspoon salt

1 teaspoon ground black pepper

1 teaspoon mustard

Directions:

Chop chives roughly.

Spray the air fryer basket tray with the olive oil.

Preheat the air fryer to 365 F.

Put the chopped chives in the air fryer basket tray.

Add the chopped green pepper and cook the vegetables for 5 minutes.

Add the ground chicken.

Chop the tomatoes into the small cubes and add them in the air fryer mixture too.

Cook the mixture for 6 minutes more.

Add the chicken stock, sliced garlic cloves, salt, ground black pepper, and mustard.

Mix well to combine.

Cook the goulash for 6 minutes more.

Nutrition:

Calories: 161

Fat: 6.1g

Carbs: 6g

Protein: 20.3g

Chicken & Turkey Meatloaf

Preparation Time: 15 minutes

Cooking Time: 25 minutes

Servings: 12

Ingredients:

3 tablespoon butter

10 oz. ground turkey

7 oz. ground chicken

1 teaspoon dried dill

½ teaspoon ground coriander

2 tablespoons almond flour

1 tablespoon minced garlic

3 oz. fresh spinach

1 teaspoon salt

1 egg

½ tablespoon paprika

1 teaspoon sesame oil

Directions:

Put the ground turkey and ground chicken in a large bowl.

Sprinkle the meat with dried dill, ground coriander, almond flour, minced garlic, salt, and paprika.

Then chop the fresh spinach and add it to the ground poultry mixture.

break the egg into the meat mixture and mix well until you get a smooth texture.

Great the air fryer basket tray with the olive oil.

Preheat the air fryer to 350 F.

Roll the ground meat mixture gently to make the flat layer.

Put the butter in the center of the meat layer.

Make the shape of the meatloaf from the ground meat mixture. Use your fingertips for this step.

Place the meatloaf in the air fryer basket tray.

Cook for 25 minutes.

When the meatloaf is cooked allow it to rest before serving.

Nutrition:

Calories: 142

Fat: 9.8 g

Carbs: 1.7g

Protein: 13g

Turkey Meatballs with Dried Dill

Preparation Time: 15 minutes

Cooking Time: 11 minutes

Servings: 9

Ingredients:

1-pound ground turkey

1 teaspoon chili flakes

¼ cup chicken stock

2 tablespoon dried dill

1 egg

1 teaspoon salt

1 teaspoon paprika

1 tablespoon coconut flour

2 tablespoons heavy cream

1 teaspoon olive oil

Directions:

in a bowl, whisk the egg with a fork.

Add the ground turkey and chili flakes.

Sprinkle the mixture with dried dill, salt, paprika, coconut flour, and mix it up.

Make the meatballs from the ground turkey mixture.

Preheat the air fryer to 360 F.

Grease the air fryer basket tray with the olive oil.

Then put the meatballs inside.

Cook the meatballs for 6 minutes – for 3 minutes on each side.

Sprinkle the meatballs with the heavy cream.

Cook the meatballs for 5 minutes more.

When the turkey meatballs are cooked – let them rest for 2-3 minutes.

Nutrition:

Calories: 124 Fat: 7.9g Carbs: 1.2g

Protein: 14.8g

<h1>CHAPTER 6:</h1>

<h1>Optavia Soup and Salads</h1>

Coconut Watercress Soup

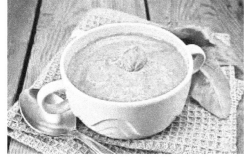

Preparation time: 10 minutes
Cooking time: 20 minutes
Servings: 4
 Ingredients:

- 1 teaspoon coconut oil
- 1 onion, diced
- ¾ cup coconut milk

Directions:

1. Melt the coconut oil in a large pot over medium-high heat. Add the onion and cook until soft, about 5 minutes, then add the peas and the water. Bring to a boil, then lower the heat and add the watercress, mint, salt, and pepper.

2. Cover and simmer for 5 minutes. Stir in the coconut milk, and purée the soup until smooth in a blender or with an immersion blender.

3. Try this soup with any other fresh, leafy green—anything from spinach to collard greens to arugula to swiss chard.

Nutrition: calories 170, fat 3, carbs 18, protein 6

Roasted Red Pepper and Butternut Squash Soup

Preparation time: 10 minutes
Cooking time: 45 minutes
Servings: 6
 Ingredients:

- 1 small butternut squash
- 1 tablespoon olive oil
- 1 teaspoon sea salt
- 2 red bell peppers
- 1 yellow onion
- 1 head garlic
- 2 cups water, or vegetable broth
- Zest and juice of 1 lime
- 1 to 2 tablespoons tahini
- Pinch cayenne pepper
- ½ teaspoon ground coriander
- ½ teaspoon ground cumin
- Toasted squash seeds (optional)

Directions:

1. Preheat the oven to 350°f.

2. Prepare the squash for roasting by cutting it in half lengthwise, scooping out the seeds, and poking some holes in the flesh with a fork. Reserve the seeds if desired.

3. Rub a small amount of oil over the flesh and skin, then rub with a bit of sea salt and put the halves skin-side down in a large baking dish. Put it in the oven while you prepare the rest of the vegetables.

4. Prepare the peppers the exact same way, except they do not need to be poked.

5. Slice the onion in half and rub oil on the exposed faces. Slice the top off the head of garlic and rub oil on the exposed flesh.

6. After the squash has cooked for 20 minutes, add the peppers, onion, and garlic, and roast for another 20 minutes. Optionally, you can toast the squash seeds by putting them in the oven in a separate baking dish 10 to 15 minutes before the vegetables are finished.

7. Keep a close eye on them. When the vegetables are cooked, take them out and let them cool before handling them. The squash will be very soft when poked with a fork.

8. Scoop the flesh out of the squash skin into a large pot (if you have an immersion blender) or into a blender.

9. Chop the pepper roughly, remove the onion skin and chop the onion roughly, and squeeze the garlic cloves out of the head, all into the pot or blender. Add the water, the lime zest and juice, and the tahini. Purée the soup, adding more water if you like, to your desired consistency. Season with the salt, cayenne, coriander, and cumin. Serve garnished with toasted squash seeds (if using).

Nutrition: calories 150, fat 3, carbs 20, protein 6

Tomato Pumpkin Soup

Preparation time: 25 minutes

Cooking time: 15 minutes

Servings: 4

Ingredients:

- 2 cups pumpkin, diced
- 1/2 cup tomato, chopped
- 1/2 cup onion, chopped

- 1 1/2 tsp curry powder
- 1/2 tsp paprika
- 2 cups vegetable stock
- 1 tsp olive oil
- 1/2 tsp garlic, minced

Directions:

1. In a saucepan, add oil, garlic, and onion and sauté for 3 minutes over medium heat.

2. Add remaining ingredients into the saucepan and bring to a boil.

3. Reduce heat and cover, and simmer for 10 minutes.

4. Puree the soup using a blender until smooth. Stir well and serve warm.

Nutrition: calories 70, fat 3, carbs 13, protein 1

Cauliflower Spinach Soup

Preparation time: 45 minutes

Cooking time: 25 minutes

Servings: 5

Ingredients:

- 1/2 cup unsweetened coconut milk
- 5 oz fresh spinach, chopped
- 5 watercress, chopped
- 8 cups vegetable stock
- 1 lb cauliflower, chopped
- Salt

Directions:

1. Add stock and cauliflower in a large saucepan and bring to a boil over medium heat for 15 minutes.

2. Add spinach and watercress and cook for another 10 minutes.

3. Remove from heat and puree the soup using a blender until smooth.

4. Add coconut milk and stir well. Season with salt. Stir well and serve hot.

Nutrition: calories 150, fat 4, carbs 8, protein 11

Avocado Mint Soup

Preparation time: 10 minutes

Cooking time: 10 minutes

Servings: 2

Ingredients:

- 1 medium avocado, peeled, pitted, and cut into pieces
- 1 cup coconut milk
- 2 romaine lettuce leaves
- 20 fresh mint leaves
- 1 tbsp fresh lime juice - 1/8 tsp salt

Directions:

1. Add all ingredients into the blender and blend until smooth. The soup should be thick, not as a puree.
2. Pour into the serving bowls and place in the refrigerator for 10 minutes.
3. Stir well and serve chilled.

Nutrition: calories 290, fat 3, carbs 18, protein 11

Creamy Squash Soup

Preparation time: 35 minutes

Cooking time: 22 minutes

Servings: 8

Ingredients:

- 3 cups butternut squash, chopped
- 1 ½ cups unsweetened coconut milk
- 1 tbsp coconut oil
- 1 tsp dried onion flakes
- 1 tbsp curry powder
- 4 cups water
- 1 garlic clove
- 1 tsp kosher salt

Directions:

1. Add squash, coconut oil, onion flakes, curry powder, water, garlic, and salt into a large saucepan. Bring to a boil over high heat.

2. Turn heat to medium and simmer for 20 minutes.
3. Puree the soup using a blender until smooth. Return soup to the saucepan and stir in coconut milk and cook for 2 minutes.
4. Stir well and serve hot.

Nutrition: calories 140, fat 2, carbs 9, protein 1

Alkaline Carrot Soup with Fresh Mushrooms

Preparation Time: *10 minutes*

Cooking Time: 20 minutes

Servings: 1-2

Ingredients:

- 4 mid-sized carrots
- 4 mid-sized potatoes
- 10 enormous new mushrooms (champignons or chanterelles)
- 1/2 white onion
- 2 tbsp. olive oil (cold squeezed, additional virgin)
- 3 cups vegetable stock
- 2 tbsp. parsley, new and cleaved
- Salt and new white pepper

Directions:

1. Wash and strip carrots and potatoes and dice them.
2. Warm up vegetable stock in a pot on medium heat. Cook carrots and potatoes for around 15 minutes. Meanwhile, finely shape onion and braise them in a container with olive oil for around 3 minutes.
3. Wash mushrooms, slice them to wanted size, and add to the container, cooking for an additional of approximately 5 minutes, blending at times. Blend carrots, vegetable stock, and potatoes, and put the substance of the skillet into the pot.

4. When nearly done, season with parsley, salt, and pepper and serve hot. Appreciate this alkalizing soup!

Nutrition: calories 176, fat 2, carbs 23, protein 9

Swiss Cauliflower-Emmenthal-Soup

Preparation Time: 10 minutes
Cooking Time: 15 minutes
Servings: 3-4
Ingredients:

- 2 cups cauliflower pieces
- 1 cup potatoes, cubed
- 2 cups vegetable stock (without yeast)
- 3 tbsp. Swiss Emmenthal cheddar, cubed
- 2 tbsp. new chives
- 1 tbsp. pumpkin seeds
- 1 touch of nutmeg and cayenne pepper

Directions:

1. Cook cauliflower and potato in vegetable stock until delicate and blend it.
2. Season the soup with nutmeg and cayenne, and possibly somewhat salt and pepper.
3. Include emmenthal cheddar and chives and mix a couple of moments until the soup is smooth and prepared to serve. Enhance it with pumpkin seeds.

Nutrition: calories 89, fat 1, carbs 18, protein 9

Cheeseburger Soup

Preparation Time: 20 minutes
Cooking Time: 25 minutes
Servings: 4
Ingredients:

- ¼ cup of chopped onion
- 1 quantity of 14.5 oz. can diced tomato
- 1 lb. of 90% lean ground beef

- ¾ cup of diced celery
- 2 teaspoon of Worcestershire sauce
- 3 cups of low sodium chicken broth
- ¼ teaspoon of salt
- 1 teaspoon of dried parsley
- 7 cups of baby spinach
- ¼ teaspoon of ground pepper
- 4 oz. of reduced-fat shredded cheddar cheese

Directions:

1. Get a large soup pot and cook the beef until it becomes brown. Add the celery, onion, and sauté until it becomes tender. Remove from the fire and drain excess liquid.
2. Stir in the broth, tomatoes, parsley, Worcestershire sauce, pepper, and salt. Cover and allow it to simmer on low heat for about 20 minutes
3. Add spinach and leave it to cook until it becomes wilted in about 1-3 minutes. Top each of your servings with 1 ounce of cheese.

Nutrition: Calories 400, Fat 5, Carbs 11, Protein 44

Chilled Avocado Tomato Soup

Preparation Time: *7 minutes*
Cooking Time: *20 minutes*
Servings: 1-2
Ingredients:

- 2 small avocados
- 2 large tomatoes
- 1 stalk of celery
- 1 small onion
- 1 clove of garlic
- Juice of 1 fresh lemon
- 1 cup of water (best: alkaline water)
- A handful of fresh lavage
- Parsley and sea salt to taste

Directions:

1. Scoop the avocados and cut all veggies into little pieces.
2. Spot all fixings in a blender and blend until smooth.
3. Serve chilled and appreciate this nutritious and sound soluble soup formula!

Nutrition: calories 210, fat 1, carbs 18, protein 9

Pumpkin and White Bean Soup with Sage

Preparation Time: 10 minutes

Cooking Time: 40 minutes

Servings: 3-4

Ingredients:

- 1 ½ pound pumpkin
- ½ pound yams
- ½ pound white beans
- 1 onion
- 2 cloves of garlic
- 1 tbsp. of cold squeezed additional virgin olive oil
- 1 tbsp. of spices (your top picks)
- 1 tbsp. of sage
- 1 ½ quart water (best: antacid water)
- A spot of ocean salt and pepper

Directions:

1. Cut the pumpkin and potatoes in shapes, cut the onion, and cut the garlic, the spices, and the sage in fine pieces.
2. Sauté the onion and also the garlic in olive oil for around two or three minutes.
3. Include the potatoes, pumpkin, spices, and sage and fry for an additional 5 minutes.
4. At that point include the water and cook for around 30 minutes (spread the pot with a top) until vegetables are delicate. Finally, include the beans and some salt and pepper. Cook for an additional 5 minutes and serve right away. Prepared!! Appreciate this antacid soup. Alkalizing tasty!

Nutrition: calories 218, fat 1, carbs 11, protein 8

Alkaline Carrot Soup with Millet

Preparation Time: 7 minutes

Cooking Time: 40 minutes

Servings: 3-4

Ingredients:

- 2 cups cauliflower pieces
- 1 cup potatoes, cubed
- 2 cups vegetable stock (without yeast)
- 3 tbsp. Swiss Emmenthal cheddar, cubed
- 2 tbsp. new chives
- 1 tbsp. pumpkin seeds
- 1 touch of nutmeg and cayenne pepper

Directions:

1. Cook cauliflower and potato in vegetable stock until delicate and blend it. Season the soup with nutmeg and cayenne, and possibly somewhat salt and pepper.
2. Include emmenthal cheddar and chives and mix a couple of moments until the soup is smooth and prepared to serve. It can be enhanced with pumpkin seeds.

Nutrition: calories 90, fat 1, carbs 18, protein 11

Alkaline Pumpkin Tomato Soup

Preparation Time: 15 minutes

Cooking Time: 30 minutes

Servings: 3-4

Ingredients:

- 1 quart of water (if accessible: soluble water)

- 400g new tomatoes, stripped and diced
- 1 medium-sized sweet pumpkin
- 5 yellow onions
- 1 tbsp. cold squeezed additional virgin olive oil
- 2 tsp. ocean salt or natural salt
- Touch of cayenne pepper
- Your preferred spices (discretionary)
- Bunch of new parsley

Directions:

1. Cut onions in little pieces and sauté with some oil in a significant pot.
2. Cut the pumpkin down the middle, at that point remove the stem and scoop out the seeds.
3. Finally, scoop out the fragile living creature and put it in the pot.
4. Include the tomatoes and the water and cook for around 20 minutes.
5. At that point, empty the soup into a food processor and blend well for a couple of moments. Sprinkle with salt, pepper, and other spices.
6. Fill bowls and trimming with new parsley. Make the most of your alkalizing soup!

Nutrition: calories 190, fat 3, carbs 18, protein 11

Alkaline Pumpkin Coconut Soup

Preparation Time: 10 minutes

Cooking Time: 15 minutes

Servings: 3-4

Ingredients:

- 2lb pumpkin
- 6 cups of water (best: soluble water delivered with a water ionizer)
- 1 cup low-fat coconut milk
- 5 ounces of potatoes
- 2 major onions
- 3 ounces leek

- 1 bunch of new parsley
- 1 touch of nutmeg
- 1 touch of cayenne pepper
- 1 tsp. ocean salt or natural salt
- 4 tbsp. cold squeezed additional virgin olive oil

Directions:

1. As a matter of first significance: cut the onions, the pumpkin, and the potatoes just as the hole into little pieces.
2. At that point, heat the olive oil in a significant pot and sauté the onions for a couple of moments.
3. At that point, include the water and heat up the pumpkin, potatoes, and the leek until delicate.
4. Include coconut milk.
5. Presently utilize a hand blender and puree for around 1 moment. The soup should turn out to be extremely velvety.
6. Season with salt, pepper, and nutmeg. Lastly, include the parsley and appreciate this alkalizing pumpkin soup hot or cold!

Nutrition: calories 90, fat 3, carbs 23, protein 1

Cold Cauliflower-Coconut Soup

Preparation Time: 7 minutes

Cooking Time: 20 minutes

Servings: 3-4

Ingredients:

- 1 pound (450g) new cauliflower
- 1 ¼ cup (300ml) unsweetened coconut milk
- 1 cup of water (best: antacid water)
- 2 tbsp. new lime juice
- 1/3 cup cold squeezed additional virgin olive oil
- 1 cup new coriander leaves, slashed
- Spot of salt and cayenne pepper

- 1 bunch of unsweetened coconut chips

Directions:

1. Steam cauliflower for around 10 minutes.

2. At that point, set up the cauliflower with coconut milk and water in a food processor and get it started until extremely smooth.

3. Include new lime squeeze, salt and pepper, a large portion of the cleaved coriander, and the oil and blend for an additional couple of moments.

4. Pour in soup bowls and embellishment with coriander and coconut chips. Appreciate!

Nutrition: calories 190, fat 1, carbs 21, protein 6

CHAPTER 7:

Optavia Smoothie Recipes

Sweet Green Smoothie

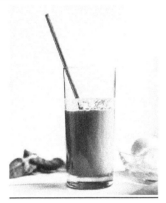

Preparation Time: 10 minutes
Cooking Time: 0 minutes
Servings: 1
Ingredients:

- 2 tablespoons flax seeds
- 1/2 cup wheatgrass - 1 mango
- 1 cup pomegranate juice

Directions:

1. Add all ingredients to the blender and blend until smooth and creamy.
2. Serve immediately and enjoy.

Nutrition: calories 177, fat 1, carbs 21, protein 5

Avocado Mango Smoothie

Preparation Time: 10 minutes
Cooking Time: 0 minutes
Servings: 2
Ingredients:

- 1 cup ice cubes

- 1/2 cup mango
- 1/2 avocado
- 1 tablespoon ginger
- 3 kale leaves
- 1 cup coconut water

Directions:

1. Toss in all your ingredients into your blender, then process until smooth.
2. Serve and Enjoy.

Nutrition: calories 290, fat 3, carbs 18, protein 11

Super Healthy Green Smoothie

Preparation Time: 10 minutes
Cooking Time: 0 minutes
Servings: 2
Ingredients:

- 1 teaspoon spirulina powder
- 1 cup coconut water
- 2 cups mixed greens
- 1 tablespoon ginger
- 4 tablespoon lemon juice
- 2 celery stalks
- 1 cup cucumber, chopped
- 1 green pear, core removed
- 1 banana

Directions:

1. Add all ingredients to the blender and blend until smooth and creamy.

2. Serve immediately and enjoy.

Nutrition: calories 161, fat 1, carbs 19, protein 7

Spinach Coconut Smoothie

Preparation Time: 10 minutes
Cooking Time: 0 minutes
Servings: 2
Ingredients:

- 2 tablespoons unsweetened coconut flakes
- 2 cups fresh pineapple
- 1/2 cup coconut water
- 1 and 1/2 cups coconut milk
- 2 cups fresh spinach

Directions:

1. Add all ingredients to the blender and blend until smooth and creamy.
2. Serve immediately and enjoy.

Nutrition: calories 290, fat 1, carbs 22, protein 8

Green Mango Smoothie

Preparation Time: 5 Minutes
Cooking Time: 0 minutes
Servings: 1
Ingredients: 2 Cups Spinach

- 1-2 Cups Coconut Water
- 2 Mangos, Ripe, Peeled & Diced

Directions:

1. Blend everything together until smooth.

Nutrition: calories 120, fat 1, carbs 5, protein 8

Chia Seed Smoothie

Preparation Time: 5 Minutes
Cooking Time: 0 minutes
Servings: 3
Ingredients:

- ¼ Teaspoon Cinnamon

- 1 Tablespoon Ginger, Fresh & Grated
- Pinch Cardamom
- 1 Tablespoon Chia Seeds
- 2 Medjool Dates, Pitted
- 1 Cup Alfalfa Sprouts
- 1 Cup Water
- 1 Banana
- ½ Cup Coconut Milk, Unsweetened

Directions:

1. Blend everything together until smooth.

Nutrition:

Calories: 412   Protein: 18.9g
Carbs: 43.8gFat: 24.8g

Mango Smoothie

Preparation Time: 5 Minutes
Cooking Time: 0 minutes
Servings: 3
Ingredients:

- 1 Carrot, Peeled & Chopped
- 1 Cup Strawberries
- 1 Cup Water
- 1 Cup Peaches, Chopped
- 1 Banana, Frozen & sliced
- 1 Cup Mango, Chopped

Directions:

1. Blend everything together until smooth.

Nutrition: calories 221, fat 1, carbs 5, protein 4

Spinach Peach Banana Smoothie

Preparation Time: 10 minutes
Cooking Time: 0 minutes
Servings: *2*
Ingredients:

- 1 cup baby spinach
- 2 cups coconut water
- 1 tablespoon agave syrup
- 2 ripe bananas

- 2 ripe peaches, pitted and chopped

Directions:

1. Add all ingredients to the blender and blend until smooth and creamy.
2. Serve immediately and enjoy.

Nutrition: calories 163, fat 1, carbs 4, protein 6

Salty Green Smoothie

Preparation Time: *10 minutes*
Cooking Time: *0 minutes*
Servings: 2
Ingredients:

- 1 cup ice cubes
- 1/4 tablespoon liquid aminos
- 1 and 1/2 tablespoon sea salt
- 2 limes, peeled and quartered
- 1 avocado, pitted and peeled
- 1 cup kale leaves
- 1 cucumber, chopped
- 2 cups tomato, chopped
- 1/4 cup water

Directions:

1. Add all ingredients to the blender and blend until smooth and creamy.
2. Serve immediately and enjoy.

Nutrition: calories 108, fat 1, carbs 1, protein 4

Watermelon Strawberry Smoothie

Preparation Time: 10 minutes
Cooking Time: 0 minutes
Servings: 2
Ingredients:

- 1 cup coconut milk yogurt
- 1/2 cup strawberries
- 2 cups fresh watermelon
- 1 banana

Directions:

1. Toss in all your ingredients into your blender, then process until smooth.
2. Serve and Enjoy.

Nutrition: calories 160, fat 1, carbs 3, protein 4

Watermelon Kale Smoothie

Preparation Time: 10 minutes
Cooking Time: 0 minutes
Servings: 2
Ingredients:

- 8 oz water
- 1 orange, peeled
- 3 cups kale, chopped
- 1 banana, peeled
- 2 cups watermelon, chopped
- 1 celery, chopped

Directions:

1. Add all ingredients to the blender and blend until smooth and creamy.
2. Serve immediately and Enjoy.

Nutrition: calories 122, fat 1, carbs 5, protein 1

Mix Berry Watermelon Smoothie

Preparation Time: *10 minutes*
Cooking Time: *0 minutes*
Servings: *2*
Ingredients: 1 cup alkaline water

- 2 fresh lemon juices
- 1/4 cup fresh mint leaves
- 1 and 1/2 cup mixed berries
- 2 cups watermelon

Directions:

1. Toss in all your ingredients into your blender, then process until smooth. Serve immediately and Enjoy.

Nutrition: calories 188, fat 1, carbs 2, protein 1

Healthy Green Smoothie

Preparation Time: 10 minutes

Cooking Time: 0 minutes

Servings: 3

Ingredients: 1 cup water

- 1 fresh lemon, peeled
- 1 avocado - 1 cucumber, peeled
- 1 cup spinach
- 1 cup ice cubes

Directions: Add all ingredients to the blender and blend until smooth and creamy. Serve immediately and enjoy.

Nutrition: Calories: 160, Fat 13, Carbs: 12, Protein 2

Apple Spinach Cucumber Smoothie

Preparation Time: 10 minutes

Cooking Time: 0 minutes

Servings: 1

Ingredients: 3/4 cup water

- 1/2 green apple, diced
- 3/4 cup spinach - 1/2 cucumber

Directions: Add all ingredients to the blender and blend until smooth and creamy. Serve immediately and enjoy.

Nutrition: calories 90, fat 1, carbs 21, protein 1

Refreshing Lime Smoothie

Preparation Time: 10 minutes

Cooking Time: 0 minutes

Servings: 2

Ingredients:

- 1 cup ice cubes

- 20 drops liquid stevia
- 2 fresh lime, peeled and halved
- 1 tablespoon lime zest, grated
- 1/2 cucumber, chopped
- 1 avocado, pitted and peeled
- 2 cups spinach
- 1 tablespoon creamed coconut
- 3/4 cup coconut water

Directions:

1. Add all ingredients to the blender and blend until smooth and creamy.
2. Serve immediately and enjoy.

Nutrition: calories 312, fat 3, carbs 28, protein 4

Broccoli Green Smoothie

Preparation Time: 10 minutes

Cooking Time: 0 minutes

Servings: 2

Ingredients:

- 1 celery, peeled and chopped
- 1 lemon, peeled
- 1 apple, diced
- 1 banana
- 1 cup spinach
- 1/2 cup broccoli

Directions:

1. Add all ingredients to the blender and blend until smooth and creamy.
2. Serve immediately and enjoy.

Nutrition: calories 121, fat 1, carbs 18, protein 1

CHAPTER 8:

Optavia Fish and Seafood Recipes

Baked Tuna 'Crab' Cakes

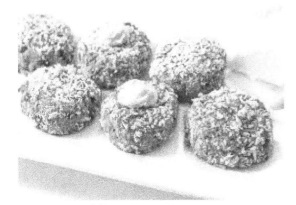

Preparation Time: 20 minutes
Cooking Time: 40 minutes
Servings: 4
Ingredients:

- 1 can chunk light tuna in water, drained and flaked
- 1 cup graham cracks crumbs
- 1 zucchini, shredded
- 1/2 green bell pepper, chopped
- 1/2 onion, finely chopped
- 1/2 cup green onions, chopped
- 2 cloves garlic, pressed or minced
- 1 teaspoon finely chopped jalapeno pepper
- 1/2 cup tofu
- 1/4 cup fat-free sour cream
- 1 lime, juiced
- 1 tablespoon dried basil
- 1 teaspoon ground black pepper
- 2 eggs

Directions:

1. Preheat oven to 350 degrees F. Line a baking sheet with aluminum foil, and spray with cooking spray.
2. Scoop up about ¼ cup of the tuna mixture and gently form it into a compact patty. And place the cakes onto the prepared baking sheet. Spray the tops of the cakes with cooking oil spray.
3. Bake in the preheated oven until the tops of the cakes are beginning to brown, about 20 minutes. Flip each cake, spray with cooking spray, and bake until the cakes are cooked through and lightly browned about 20 more minutes.

Nutrition: Calories 63, fat 24, carbs 18, Protein 35,

Baked Fennel & Garlic Sea Bass

Preparation time: 5 minutes
Cooking time: 15 minutes
Servings: 2
Ingredients:

- 1 lemon
- ½ sliced fennel bulb
- 6 oz. sea bass fillets
- 1 tsp. black pepper
- 2 garlic cloves

Direction:

1. Preheat the oven to 375°F/Gas Mark 5.

2. Sprinkle black pepper over the Sea Bass.

3. Slice the fennel bulb and garlic cloves.

4. Add 1 salmon fillet and half the fennel and garlic to one sheet of baking paper or tin foil.

5. Squeeze in 1/2 lemon juices.

6. Repeat for the other fillet.

7. Fold and add to the oven for 12-15 minutes or until fish is thoroughly cooked through.

8. Meanwhile, add boiling water to your couscous, cover, and allow to steam.

9. Serve with your choice of rice or salad.

Nutrition: calories 221, fat 8, carbs 4, protein 14

Lemon, Garlic & Cilantro Tuna and Rice

Preparation time: 5 minutes

Cooking time: 0 minutes

Servings: 2

Ingredients:

- ½ cup arugula
- 1 tbsp. extra virgin olive oil
- 1 cup cooked rice
- 1 tsp. black pepper
- ¼ finely diced red onion
- 1 juiced lemon
- 3 oz. canned tuna
- 2 tbsps. Chopped fresh cilantro

Directions:

1. Mix the olive oil, pepper, cilantro, and red onion in a bowl.

2. Stir in the tuna, cover, and leave in the fridge for as long as possible (if you can), or serve immediately.

3. When ready to eat, serve up with the cooked rice and arugula!

Nutrition: calories 320, fat 7, carbs 3, protein 42

Cod & Green Bean Risotto

Preparation time: 4 minutes

Cooking time: 40 minutes

Servings: 2

Ingredients:

- ½ cup arugula
- 1 finely diced white onion
- 4 oz. cod fillet
- 1 cup white rice
- 2 lemon wedges
- 1 cup boiling water
- ¼ tsp. black pepper
- 1 cup low sodium chicken broth
- 1 tbsp. extra virgin olive oil
- ½ cup green beans

Directions:

1. Heat the oil in a large pan on medium heat.

2. Sauté the chopped onion for 5 minutes until soft before adding in the rice and stirring for 1-2 minutes.

3. Combine the broth with boiling water.

4. Add half of the liquid to the pan and stir slowly.

5. Slowly add the rest of the liquid whilst continuously stirring for up to 20-30 minutes.

6. Stir in the green beans to the risotto.

7. Place the fish on top of the rice, cover, and steam for 10 minutes.

8. Ensure the water does not dry out and keep topping up until the rice is cooked thoroughly.

9. Use your fork to break up the fish fillets and stir into the rice.

10. Sprinkle with freshly ground pepper to serve and a squeeze of fresh lemon.

11. Garnish with the lemon wedges and serve with the arugula.

Nutrition: calories 219, fat 18, carbs 3, protein 40

Sardine Fish Cakes

Preparation Time: 10 minutes
Cooking Time: 10 minutes
Servings: 4
Ingredients:

- 11 oz sardines, canned, drained
- 1/3 cup shallot, chopped
- 1 teaspoon chili flakes
- ½ teaspoon salt
- 2 tablespoon wheat flour, whole grain
- 1 egg, beaten
- 1 tablespoon chives, chopped
- 1 teaspoon olive oil
- 1 teaspoon butter

Directions:

1. Put the butter in the skillet and melt it.
2. Add shallot and cook it until translucent.
3. After this, transfer the shallot to the mixing bowl.
4. Add sardines, chili flakes, salt, flour, egg, chives, and mix up until smooth with the help of the fork.
5. Make the medium size cakes and place them in the skillet.
6. Add olive oil.
7. Roast the fish cakes for 3 minutes from each side over medium heat.
8. Dry the cooked fish cakes with a paper towel if needed and transfer to the serving plates.

Nutrition: calories 356, fat 23, carbs 1, protein 38

Savory Cilantro Salmon

Preparation Time: 10 minutes
Cooking Time: 30 minutes
Servings: 4
Ingredients:

2 tablespoons of fresh lime or lemon
4 cups of fresh cilantro, divided
2 tablespoon of hot red pepper sauce
½ teaspoon of salt. Divided
1 teaspoon of cumin
4, 7 oz. of salmon filets
½ cup of (4 oz.) water
2 cups of sliced red bell pepper
2 cups of sliced yellow bell pepper
2 cups of sliced green bell pepper
Cooking spray
½ teaspoon of pepper

Directions:

Get a blender or food processor and combine half of the cilantro, lime juice or lemon, cumin, hot red pepper sauce, water, and salt; then puree until they become smooth. Transfer the marinade gotten into a large re-sealable plastic bag.

Add salmon to marinade. Seal the bag, squeeze out air that might have been trapped inside, turn to coat salmon. Refrigerate for about 1 hour, turning as often as possible.

Now, after marinating, preheat your oven to about 4000F. Arrange the pepper slices in a single layer in a slightly-greased, medium-sized square baking dish. Bake it for 20 minutes, turn the pepper slices once. Drain your salmon and do away with the marinade. Crust the upper part of the salmon with the remaining chopped, fresh cilantro. Place salmon on the top of the pepper slices and bake for about 12-14 minutes until you observe that the fish flakes easily when it is being tested with a fork

Enjoy

Nutrition: Calories: 350 Carbohydrate: 15 g Protein: 42 g Fat: 13 g

Cajun Catfish

Preparation Time: 10 minutes
Cooking Time: 10 minutes
Servings: 4
Ingredients:

- 16 oz catfish steaks (4 oz each fish steak)

- 1 tablespoon cajun spices
- 1 egg, beaten
- 1 tablespoon sunflower oil

Directions:

1. Pour sunflower oil into the skillet and preheat it until shimmering.
2. Meanwhile, dip every catfish steak in the beaten egg and coat it in Cajun spices.
3. Place the fish steaks in the hot oil and roast them for 4 minutes from each side.
4. The cooked catfish steaks should have a light brown crust.

Nutrition: calories 435, fat 7, carbs 8, protein 49

4-Ingredients Salmon Fillet

Preparation Time: 5 minutes
Cooking Time: 25 minutes
Servings: 1
Ingredients:

- 4 oz salmon fillet
- ½ teaspoon salt
- 1 teaspoon sesame oil
- ½ teaspoon sage

Directions:

1. Rub the fillet with salt and sage.
2. Place the fish in the tray and sprinkle it with sesame oil.
3. Cook the fish for 25 minutes at 365F.
4. Flip the fish carefully onto another side after 12 minutes of cooking.

Nutrition: calories 190, fat 11, carbs 4, protein 22

Spanish Cod in Sauce

Preparation Time: 10 minutes
Cooking Time: 5.5 hours
Servings: 2
Ingredients:

- 1 teaspoon tomato paste

- 1 teaspoon garlic, diced
- 1 white onion, sliced
- 1 jalapeno pepper, chopped
- 1/3 cup chicken stock
- 7 oz Spanish cod fillet
- 1 teaspoon paprika
- 1 teaspoon salt

Directions:

1. Pour chicken stock into the saucepan.
2. Add tomato paste and mix up the liquid until homogenous.
3. Add garlic, onion, jalapeno pepper, paprika, and salt.
4. Bring the liquid to a boil and then simmer it.
5. Chop the cod fillet and add it to the tomato liquid.
6. Close the lid and simmer the fish for 10 minutes over low heat.
7. Serve the fish in the bowls with tomato sauce.

Nutrition: calories 112, fat 1, carbs 5, protein 18

Fish Shakshuka

Preparation Time: 5 minutes
Cooking Time: 15 minutes
Servings: 5
Ingredients:

- 5 eggs
- 1 cup tomatoes, chopped
- 3 bell peppers, chopped
- 1 tablespoon butter
- 1 teaspoon tomato paste
- 1 teaspoon chili pepper
- 1 teaspoon salt
- 1 tablespoon fresh dill
- 5 oz cod fillet, chopped
- 1 tablespoon scallions, chopped

Directions:

1. Melt butter in the skillet and add chili pepper, bell peppers, and tomatoes.
2. Sprinkle the vegetables with scallions, dill, salt, and chili pepper. Simmer them for 5 minutes.
3. After this, add chopped cod fillet and mix up well.
4. Close the lid and simmer the ingredients for 5 minutes over medium heat. Then crack the eggs over the fish and close the lid. Cook shakshuka with the closed lid for 5 minutes.

Nutrition: calories 143, fat 3, carbs 8, protein 12

Salmon Baked in Foil with Fresh Thyme

Preparation Time: 10 minutes
Cooking Time: 30 minutes
Servings: 4
Ingredients:

- 4 fresh thyme sprig
- 4 garlic cloves, peeled, roughly chopped
- 16 oz salmon fillets (4 oz each fillet)
- ½ teaspoon salt
- ½ teaspoon ground black pepper
- 4 tablespoons cream
- 4 teaspoons butter
- ¼ teaspoon cumin seeds

Directions:

1. Line the baking tray with foil.
2. Sprinkle the fish fillets with salt, ground black pepper, cumin seeds, and arrange them in the tray with oil.
3. Add thyme sprig on the top of every fillet.
4. Then add cream, butter, and garlic.
5. Bake the fish for 30 minutes at 345F.

Nutrition: calories 189, fat 11, carbs 2, protein 22

Poached Halibut in Orange Sauce
Preparation Time: 10 minutes
Cooking Time: 10 minutes
Servings: 4
Ingredients:

- 1-pound halibut
- 1/3 cup butter
- 1 rosemary sprig
- ½ teaspoon ground black pepper
- 1 teaspoon salt
- 1 teaspoon honey
- ¼ cup of orange juice
- 1 teaspoon cornstarch

Directions:

1. Put butter in the saucepan and melt it.
2. Add rosemary sprig.
3. Sprinkle the halibut with salt and ground black pepper.
4. Put the fish in the boiling butter and poach it for 4 minutes.
5. Meanwhile, pour orange juice into the skillet. Add honey and bring the liquid to a boil.
6. Add cornstarch and whisk until the liquid starts to be thick.
7. Then remove it from the heat.
8. Transfer the poached halibut to the plate and cut it on 4.
9. Place every fish serving on the serving plate and top with orange sauce.

Nutrition: calories 349, fat 4, carbs 6, protein 19

Fishen Papillote

Preparation Time: 15 minutes
Cooking Time: 20 minutes
Servings: 3
Ingredients:

- 10 oz snapper fillet
- 1 tablespoon fresh dill, chopped

- 1 white onion, peeled, sliced
- ½ teaspoon tarragon
- 1 tablespoon olive oil
- 1 teaspoon salt
- ½ teaspoon hot pepper
- 2 tablespoons sour cream

Directions:

1. Make the medium size packets from parchment and arrange them in the baking tray.
2. Cut the snapper fillet into 3 and sprinkle them with salt, tarragon, and hot pepper.
3. Put the fish fillets in the parchment packets.
4. Then top the fish with olive oil, sour cream, sliced onion, and fresh dill.
5. Bake the fish for 20 minutes at 355F.

Nutrition: Calories 204, Fat 8g, Carbohydrate 4.6g, Protein 27g

Tuna Casserole

Preparation Time: 15 minutes

Cooking Time: 35 minutes

Servings: 4

Ingredients:

- ½ cup Cheddar cheese, shredded
- 2 tomatoes, chopped
- 7 oz tuna filet, chopped
- 1 teaspoon ground coriander
- ½ teaspoon salt
- 1 teaspoon olive oil
- ½ teaspoon dried oregano

Directions:

1. Brush the casserole mold with olive oil.
2. Mix up together chopped tuna fillet with dried oregano and ground coriander.
3. Place the fish in the mold and flatten well to get the layer.

4. Then add chopped tomatoes and shredded cheese.
5. Cover the casserole with foil and secure the edges.
6. Bake the meal for 35 minutes at 355F.

Nutrition: Calories 260, Fat 21, Carbohydrate 3, Protein 14

Oregano Salmon with Crunchy Crust

Preparation Time: 10 minutes

Cooking Time: 2 hours

Servings: 2

Ingredients:

- 8 oz salmon fillet
- 2 tablespoons panko breadcrumbs
- 1 oz Parmesan, grated
- 1 teaspoon dried oregano
- 1 teaspoon sunflower oil

Directions:

1. In the mixing bowl, combine together panko breadcrumbs, Parmesan, and dried oregano.
2. Sprinkle the salmon with olive oil and coat in the breadcrumb's mixture.
3. After this, line the baking tray with baking paper.
4. Place the salmon in the tray and transfer in the preheated to the 385F oven.
5. Bake the salmon for 25 minutes.

Nutrition: Calories 245, Fat 8, Carbohydrate 6, Protein 6

Ginger Shrimp with Snow Peas

Preparation Time: 20 minutes

Cooking Time: 12 minutes

Servings: 4

Ingredients:

- 2 tablespoons of extra-virgin olive oil
- 1 tablespoon of minced peeled fresh ginger

- 2 cups of snow peas
- 1½ cups of frozen baby peas
- 3 tablespoons of water
- 1 pound of medium shrimp, shelled and deveined
- 2 tablespoons of low-sodium soy sauce
- ⅛ teaspoon of freshly ground black pepper

Directions:

1. Using a large wok, heat the olive oil over medium heat.
2. Add the ginger and stir-fry for 1 to 2 minutes until the ginger is fragrant.
3. Add the snow peas and stir-fry for 2 to 3 minutes until they are tender-crisp.
4. Add the baby peas and the water and stir. Cover the wok and steam for 2 to 3 minutes or until the vegetables are tender.
5. Stir in the shrimp and stir-fry for 3 to 4 minutes, or until the shrimp have curled and turned pink.
6. Add the soy sauce and pepper; stir and serve.

Nutrition: Calories: *237* Fat: *7,* Carbs: *12,* Protein: *32*

Fish Chili with Lentils

Preparation Time: 10 minutes
Cooking Time: 30 minutes
Servings: 4
Ingredients:

- 1 red pepper, chopped
- 1 yellow onion, diced
- 1 teaspoon ground black pepper
- 1 teaspoon butter
- 1 jalapeno pepper, chopped
- ½ cup lentils
- 3 cups chicken stock
- 1 teaspoon salt
- 1 tablespoon tomato paste

- 1 teaspoon chili pepper
- 3 tablespoons fresh cilantro, chopped
- 8 oz cod, chopped

Directions:

1. Place butter, red pepper, onion, and ground black pepper in the saucepan.
2. Roast the vegetables for 5 minutes over medium heat.
3. Then add chopped jalapeno pepper, lentils, and chili pepper.
4. Mix up the mixture well and add chicken stock and tomato paste.
5. Stir until homogenous. Add cod.
6. Close the lid and cook chili for 20 minutes over medium heat.

Nutrition: calories 321, fat 21, carbs 18, protein 34

Chili Mussels

Preparation Time: 7 minutes
Cooking Time: 10 minutes
Servings: 4
Ingredients:

- 1-pound mussels
- 1 chili pepper, chopped
- 1 cup chicken stock
- ½ cup milk
- 1 teaspoon olive oil
- 1 teaspoon minced garlic
- 1 teaspoon ground coriander
- ½ teaspoon salt
- 1 cup fresh parsley, chopped
- 4 tablespoons lemon juice

Directions:

1. Pour milk into the saucepan.
2. Add chili pepper, chicken stock, olive oil, minced garlic, ground coriander, salt, and lemon juice.
3. Bring the liquid to a boil and add mussels.

4. Boil the mussel for 4 minutes or until they will open the shells.
5. Then add chopped parsley and mix up the meal well.
6. Remove it from the heat.

Nutrition: Calories: 355 Carbs: 9g Fat: 29g Protein: 17g

Fried Scallops in Heavy Cream

Preparation Time: 10 minutes
Cooking Time: 7 minutes
Servings: 4
Ingredients:

- ½ cup heavy cream
- 1 teaspoon fresh rosemary
- ½ teaspoon dried cumin
- ½ teaspoon garlic, diced
- 8 oz bay scallops
- 1 teaspoon olive oil
- ½ teaspoon salt
- ¼ teaspoon chili flakes

Directions:

1. Preheat olive oil in the skillet until hot.
2. Then sprinkle scallops with salt, chili flakes, and dried cumin and place in the hot oil.
3. Add fresh rosemary and diced garlic.
4. Roast the scallops for 2 minutes from each side.
5. After this, add heavy cream and bring the mixture to a boil. Boil it for 1 minute.

Nutrition: calories 151, fat 19, carbs 4, protein 22

Lettuce Seafood Wraps

Preparation Time: 10 minutes
Cooking Time: 0 minutes
Servings: 6
Ingredients:

- 6 lettuce leaves

- 8 oz salmon, canned
- 4 oz crab meat, canned
- 1 cucumber
- 2 tablespoons Plain yogurt
- ½ teaspoon minced garlic
- 1 tablespoon fresh dill, chopped
- ¼ teaspoon tarragon

Directions:

1. Mash the salmon and crab meat with the help of the fork.
2. Then add Plain yogurt, minced garlic, fresh dill, and tarragon.
3. Grate the cucumber and add it to the seafood mixture. Mix up well.
4. Fill the lettuce leaves with the cooked mixture.

Nutrition: calories 344, fat 1, carbs 18, protein 1

Mango Tilapia Fillets

Preparation Time: 10 minutes
Cooking Time: 15 minutes
Servings: 4
Ingredients:

- ¼ cup coconut flakes
- 5 oz mango, peeled
- 1/3 cup shallot, chopped
- 1 teaspoon ground turmeric
- 1 cup of water
- 1 bay leaf
- 12 oz tilapia fillets
- 1 chili pepper, chopped
- 1 tablespoon coconut oil
- ½ teaspoon salt
- 1 teaspoon paprika

Directions:

1. Blend together coconut flakes, mango, shallot, ground turmeric, and water.
2. After this, melt coconut oil in the saucepan.

3. Sprinkle the tilapia fillets with salt and paprika.
4. Then place them in the hot coconut oil and roast for 1 minute from each side.
5. Add chili pepper, bay leaf, and blended mango mixture.
6. Close the lid and cook the fish for 10 minutes over medium heat.

Nutrition: calories 342, fat 1, carbs 18, protein 23

Lemon Butter Fillet

Preparation Time: 20 minutes
Cooking Time: 30 minutes
Servings: 5
Ingredients:

- 1/2 cup butter
- 1 lemon, juiced
- 1 teaspoon ground black pepper
- 1/2 teaspoon dried basil
- 3 cloves garlic, minced
- 6 (4 ounce) fillets cod
- 2 tablespoons lemon pepper

Directions:

1. Preheat oven to 350 degrees F.
2. Melt the butter in a medium saucepan over medium heat. Bring to a boil.
3. Arrange cod fillets in a single layer on a medium baking sheet. Cover with 1/2 the butter mixture, and sprinkle with lemon pepper. Cover with foil.

Nutrition: calories 169, fat 4, carbs 5, protein 33

Fish Soup

Preparation Time: 10 minutes
Cooking Time: 30 minutes
Servings: 5
Ingredients:

- 1/2 onion, chopped
- 1 clove garlic, minced

- 1 tablespoon chili powder
- 1 1/2 cups chicken broth
- 1 teaspoon ground cumin
- 1/2 cup chopped green bell pepper
- 1/2 cup shrimp
- 1/2 pound cod fillets
- 3/4 cup plain yogurt

Directions:

1. Spray a large saucepan with the cooking spray over medium-high heat. Add the onions and sauté, stirring often, for about 5 minutes. Add the garlic and chili powder and sauté for 2 more minutes.
2. Then add the chicken broth and cumin, stirring well. Bring to a boil, reduce heat to low, cover and simmer for 20 minutes.
3. Next, add green bell pepper, shrimp, and cod. Return to a boil, then reduce heat to low, cover, and simmer for another 5 minutes. Gradually stir in the yogurt until heated through.

Nutrition: calories 390, fat 5, carbs 28, protein 41

Cod Egg Sandwich

Preparation Time: 10 minutes
Cooking Time: 10 minutes
Servings: 2
Ingredients:

- 2 (5 ounce) can cod, drained 6 hard-cooked eggs, peeled and chopped
- 2 cups chopped celery
- 2 tablespoons mayonnaise
- Pepper to taste
- 8 slices white bread

Directions:

1. In a medium bowl, stir together the cod, eggs, celery, and mayonnaise. Season with pepper to taste. Place half of the

mixture onto 1 slice of bread and the other half on another slice of bread.

2. Top with remaining slices of bread. Serve.

Nutrition: calories 110, fat 16, carbs 18, protein 43

Tuna Mushroom Casserole
Preparation Time: 10 minutes
Cooking Time: 53 minutes
Servings: 3
Ingredients:

- 2 cups macaroni
- 2 (5 ounce) cans tuna, drained
- 1 (10 ounce) can mushrooms, drained
- 1 cup water
- 1 1/3 cups soy milk
- 1/4 teaspoon freshly ground black pepper
- 1 cup dry white bread crumbs
- 3 tablespoons melted butter
- 2 teaspoons dried thyme, crushed

Directions:

1. In a mixing bowl, combine bread crumbs, butter, and thyme. Mix well. Sprinkle over the top of the tuna mixture.
2. Bake uncovered in a preheated oven until bubbling and golden brown, about 40 minutes.

Nutrition: calories 422, fat 12, carbs 18, protein 1

Ginger and Lime Salmon
Preparation Time: 15 minutes
Cooking Time: 15 minutes
Servings: 2
Ingredients:

- 1 (1 1/2-pound) salmon fillet
- 1 tablespoon olive oil

- 1 teaspoon oregano
- 1 teaspoon ground black pepper
- 1 (1 inch) piece fresh ginger root, peeled and thinly sliced
- 6 cloves garlic, minced
- 1 lime, thinly sliced

Directions:

1. Season with oregano and black pepper.
2. Broil salmon until hot and beginning to turn opaque, about 10 minutes; watch carefully.
3. If the broiler has a High setting, turn the broiler to that setting and continue broiling until salmon is cooked through and flakes easily with a fork, 5 to 10 more minutes.

Nutrition: calories 121, fat 32, carbs 18, protein 43

Lemon Rosemary Salmon with Garlic
Preparation Time: 15 minutes
Cooking Time: 35 minutes
Servings: 3
Ingredients:

- 1/4 cup butter, melted
- 1/4 cup white wine
- 1 lemon, juiced
- 5 cloves garlic, chopped
- 1 bunch fresh rosemary, stems trimmed
- 1 (1 pound) salmon fillet

Directions:

1. Preheat oven to 375 degrees F. Mix butter, white wine, lemon juice, and garlic together in a small bowl.
2. Bake for 25 minutes.

Nutrition: calories 324, fat 12, carbs 1, protein 41

Lemon-Pepper Salmon with Couscous

Preparation Time: 10 minutes

Cooking Time: 20 minutes

Servings: 5

Ingredients:

- 2 tablespoons olive oil
- 4 (4 ounce) salmon steaks
- 1 teaspoon minced garlic
- 1 tablespoon lemon pepper
- 1/4 cup water
- 1 cup chopped fresh cilantro
- 2 cups boiling water
- 1 cup uncooked couscous

Directions:

1. Heat the olive oil in a large skillet over medium heat. Place salmon in the skillet, and season with garlic and lemon pepper. Pour 1/4 cup water around salmon. Place cilantro in the skillet. Cover and cook for 15 minutes, or until fish is easily flaked with a fork.

2. Bring 2 cups of water to boil in a pot. Remove from heat, and mix in couscous. Cover and let sit for 5 minutes. Serve the cooked salmon over couscous, and drizzle with sauce from skillet.

Nutrition: calories 121, fat 19, carbs 18, protein 48

CHAPTER 9:

Optavia Poultry Recipes

Sweet and Spicy Firecracker Chicken

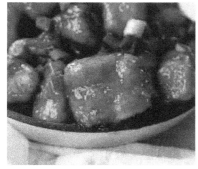

Preparation time: 9 minutes

Cooking Time: 35 minutes

Servings: 4

Ingredients:

- 1/2 cup packed light brown sugar
- 1/3 cup buffalo sauce
- 1 tablespoon apple cider vinegar
- salt
- 1/4 teaspoon red pepper flakes
- 1 lb. boneless skinless chicken breast
- 1/2 cup cornstarch
- 2 large eggs

Directions:

1. Start by cutting the chicken breast into 1-inch cubes.
2. Mix buffalo sauce in a bowl, apple cider vinegar, salt, and red pepper flakes.
3. Place the cornstarch in a plastic container or bag.
4. Beat the eggs in a bowl.
5. Toss the chicken in the cornstarch, then dip it in the egg.
6. Cook chicken in your air fryer at 360F for about 5 minutes; the chicken does not need to be fully cooked, only crisp on the outside.
7. Place the chicken in a baking pan and pour the buffalo sauce mixture over it. Return to the air fryer.
8. Continue to bake at 350F for 30 minutes.

Nutrition: Calories: 385, Fat: 7, Carbs: 38, Protein: 40

Fried Chicken Livers

Preparation time: 9 minutes

Cooking Time: 10 minutes

Servings: 4

Ingredients:

- 1 lb. chicken livers
- 1 cup flour
- 1/2 cup cornmeal
- 2 teaspoons herbs Provence
- 3 eggs
- 2 tablespoons milk

Directions:

1. Clean and rinse the livers, pat dry.
2. Beat eggs in a shallow bowl and mix in milk.
3. In another bowl, combine flour, cornmeal, and seasoning, mixing until even.
4. Dip the livers in the egg mix, then toss them in the flour mix.

5. Air fry at 375F for 10 minutes. Toss at least once halfway through.

Nutrition: Calories: 409, Fat: 11, Carbs: 37, Protein: 36

Turkey with Maple Mustard Glaze

Preparation time: 13 minutes

Cooking Time: minutes

Servings: 4

Ingredients:

- 2 teaspoons olive oil
- 3 lbs. whole turkey breast
- 1 teaspoon dried thyme
- 1/2 teaspoon dried sage
- 1/2 teaspoon smoked paprika
- 1 teaspoon salt
- 1/2 teaspoon black pepper
- 1/4 cup maple syrup
- 2 tablespoons Dijon mustard
- 1 tablespoon butter

Directions:

1. Preheat the air fryer to 350°F. Brush the entire turkey breast with olive oil.
2. Combine dry seasonings and toss to mix.
3. Rub the seasonings over the turkey and put it in the air fryer, frying for 25 minutes.
4. Turn it on one side and fry for another 12 minutes. Turn it on the other side, then cook for 11 more minutes.
5. Melt the butter in a bowl and mix in syrup and mustard.
6. Return the turkey to its upright position and brush the syrup mix over the turkey.
7. Cook for 5 more minutes before serving. Enjoy!!

Nutrition: Calories: 404, Fat: 8, Carbs: 14, Protein: 58

Chicken Parmesan

Preparation time: 9 minutes

Cooking Time: 10 minutes

Servings: 4

Ingredients:

- 2 (8 ounce) chicken breast
- 6 tablespoons seasoned breadcrumbs
- 2 tablespoons parmesan cheese
- 1 tablespoon olive oil
- 6 tablespoons mozzarella cheese
- 1/2 cup marinara sauce
- Cooking spray

Directions:

1. Cut the chicken in half vertically to create 4 breasts.
2. Mix the breadcrumbs and parmesan together in a bowl.
3. Brush the chicken with olive oil.
4. Press the chicken into the breadcrumb mix.
5. Preheat the air fryer to 360°F.
6. Place 2 chicken breasts in the basket and spray with cooking spray.
7. Cook for 6 minutes.
8. Flip the chicken and top with 1 tablespoon marinara and 1 - 1/2 tablespoons mozzarella.
9. Cook for 3 more minutes, then repeat with the other 2 breasts.

Nutrition: Calories: 250, Fat: 14, Carbs: 11, Protein: 18

Chicken Fajita Roll Ups

Preparation time: 25 minutes

Cooking Time: 12 minutes

Servings: 6

Ingredients:

- 3 chicken breasts
- 1/2 red, green, and yellow bell pepper
- 1/2 red onion

- 2 teaspoons paprika
- 1 teaspoon garlic powder
- 1 teaspoon cumin powder
- 1/2 teaspoon cayenne
- 1/2 teaspoon oregano
- Salt and pepper, to taste
- Cooking spray
- Toothpicks

Directions:

1. Cut the bell pepper halves vertically into thin strips.
2. Mix together all of your spices.
3. Cut into half each chicken breast through the middle.
4. Pound each breast half flat.
5. Season both sides of each piece of chicken with the spice blend.
6. Place 2 bell pepper strips of each color and a few pieces of onion in the center of each piece of chicken.
7. Roll the chicken up around the peppers and onions and use 1 or 2 toothpicks to hold the roll up shut.
8. Preheat your air fryer to 390°F.
9. Spray each roll up with cooking spray and cook 3 at a time for 12 minutes.

Nutrition: Calories: 70, Fat: 2, Carbs: 3, Protein: 11

Tandoori Chicken

Preparation time: 25 minutes

Cooking Time: 30 minutes

Servings: 4

Ingredients:

- 4 chicken legs
- 3 teaspoons ginger paste
- 3 teaspoons garlic paste
- Salt to taste
- 3 tablespoons lemon juice
- 2 tablespoon tandoori masala powder

- 1 teaspoon roasted cumin powder
- 1 teaspoon garam masala powder
- 2 teaspoons red chili powder
- 1 teaspoon turmeric powder
- 4 tablespoons hung curd
- 2 teaspoons kasoori methi
- 1 teaspoon black pepper
- 2 teaspoons coriander powder

Directions:

1. Wash the chicken legs and cut a few slits in each one. Mix ginger paste, garlic paste, and salt together.
2. Put the chicken in a bowl and coat with the ginger paste mix. Set the chicken in the fridge for 15 minutes.
3. While the chicken marinates, mix all the other ingredients together.
4. Pour the marinade over the chicken and return to the fridge for at least 10 hours.
5. Preheat the air fryer to 360°F. Cook the chicken for 30 minutes, turning halfway through.

Nutrition: Calories: 186, Fat: 12, Carbs: 5, Protein: 13

Crispy Coconut Chicken

Preparation time: 15 minutes

Cooking Time: 15 minutes

Servings: 4

Ingredients:

- 1/2 cup cornstarch
- 1/4 Tbs. salt
- 1/8 teaspoon pepper
- 3 eggs
- 2 cups sweetened coconut flakes
- 2 cups unsweetened coconut flakes
- 4 medium boneless chicken breasts

Directions:

1. Beat the eggs and cut the chicken into strips.
2. Mix cornstarch, salt, and pepper in a separate bowl.
3. Place your sweetened and unsweetened coconut in a third shallow bowl or plate; mix well.
4. Roll the chicken in the cornstarch mix.
5. Dip the chicken in the egg, then roll it in coconut.
6. Preheat the air fryer to 360°F.
7. Cook for 15 minutes, flipping halfway through.

Nutrition: Calories: 452, Fat: 30, Carbs: 27, Protein: 19

Homemade Chicken Nuggets

Preparation time: 10 minutes
Cooking Time: 10 minutes
Servings: 4
Ingredients:

- 2 (8 ounce) skinless boneless chicken breasts, cut into nugget sized pieces
- Salt and pepper, to taste
- 2 teaspoons olive oil
- 6 tablespoons Italian seasoned breadcrumbs
- 2 tablespoons panko breadcrumbs
- 2 tablespoons parmesan cheese
- Olive oil spray

Directions:

1. Put chicken, olive oil, salt, and pepper in a bowl and toss to coat.
2. Mix the breadcrumbs and parmesan together in a bowl.
3. Toss the chicken in the breadcrumb mixture.
4. Place the chicken in the basket and spray with olive oil spray.
5. Preheat the air fryer to 390°F.

6. Cook for 10 minutes, tossing halfway through.

Nutrition: Calories: 338, Fat: 9, Carbs: 9, Protein: 50

Buffalo Chicken Meatballs

Preparation time: 10 minutes
Cooking Time: 10 minutes
Servings: 4
Ingredients:

- 1 lb. ground chicken
- 4 garlic cloves
- 1 package ranch seasoning
- 1 cup seasoned breadcrumbs
- 1 cup hot sauce
- 1 cup ranch dressing
- 1/2 cup blue cheese crumbles

Directions:

1. Mince the garlic.
2. Combine garlic, ranch seasoning, and breadcrumbs in a large bowl.
3. Add the chicken and knead the ingredients together.
4. Roll into small balls.
5. Cook for 360°F for 5 minutes using the air fryer.
6. Toss the meatballs in the hot sauce and cook up to another 5 minutes.
7. Mix together ranch and blue cheese crumbles.
8. Drizzle ranch mix over meatballs before serving.

Nutrition: Calories: 326, Fat: 13, Carbs: 10, Protein: 37

Chicken Wontons

Preparation time: 25 minutes
Cooking Time: 12 minutes
Servings: 4
Ingredients:

- 1 cup all-purpose flour

- 1/4 lb. boneless skinless chicken breast
- 1 egg
- 1 green onion
- 1 tablespoon French beans
- 1 tablespoon carrots
- 1/2 teaspoon pepper powder
- 1/4 teaspoon soy sauce
- 1/2 teaspoon cornstarch
- 1 teaspoon sesame seed oil

Directions:

1. Finely dice all of your vegetables, beans, and chicken into the smallest pieces possible.
2. Mix flour, salt, and a little hot water to create a stiff dough. Cover and set aside.
3. Beat the egg in a large bowl. Add all other ingredients, except for the sesame seed oil, to the egg bowl and mix well.
4. Add the sesame seed oil to the mix and mix again.
5. Roll your dough flat and use a cookie cutter to cut it into circles about 6 inches in diameter. You can also use pre-made wonton wrappers.
6. Preheat the air fryer to 360°F. Scoop a little mixture into the center of each circle.
7. Use your fingers to wet the edges of the circles. Fold them over the stuffing and press to close. Cook in the fryer for 12 minutes, flipping them after 7 minutes.

Nutrition: Calories: 185, Fat: 3, Carbs: 27, Protein: 11

Chicken Kabobs

Preparation time: 15 minutes
Cooking Time: 20 minutes
Servings: 2
Ingredients:

- 2 chicken breasts

- 1/3 cup honey
- 1/3 cup soy sauce
- Sesame seeds
- 6 mushrooms
- 1 each- red, yellow, and green bell pepper
- Cooking spray
- Salt to taste

Directions:

1. Cut the chicken breast into cubes.
2. Spray the cubes with cooking spray and season with salt
3. Transfer to a bowl and mix chicken with honey, soy sauce, and sesame seeds. Cut mushrooms in half.
4. Preheat your air fryer to 340°F.
5. Add chicken, peppers, and mushrooms onto the skewers, alternating each one until the skewers are full.
6. Cook in the air fryer for 20 minutes, turning the kabobs at the halfway mark.

Nutrition: Calories: 377, Fat: 3, Carbs: 65, Protein: 27

Perfect Juicy Chicken Breast

Preparation Time: 15 minutes
Cooking Time: 25 minutes
Servings: 8
Ingredients:

- 4 chicken breasts, skinless and boneless
- 1 tbsp. olive oil

For rub:

- 1 tsp. garlic powder
- 1 tsp. onion powder
- 4 tsp. brown sugar
- 4 tsp. paprika
- 1 tsp. black pepper
- 1 tsp. salt

Directions:

1. Insert wire rack in rack position 6. Select bake, set temperature 390 F, timer for 30 minutes. Press start to preheat the oven.
2. Brush chicken breasts with olive oil. In a small bowl, mix together rub ingredients and rub all over chicken breasts.
3. Arrange chicken breasts on a roasting pan and bake for 12-15 minutes or until internal temperature reaches 165 F.
4. Serve and enjoy.

Nutrition: Calories 165, Fat 7, Carbs 3, Protein 21

Crispy & Tasty Chicken Breast

Preparation Time: 15 minutes
Cooking Time: 35 minutes
Servings: 4
Ingredients:

- 4 chicken breasts, skinless and boneless
- 1/2 cup butter, cut into pieces
- 1 cup cracker crumbs
- 3 eggs, lightly beaten
- Pepper
- Salt

Directions:

1. Insert wire rack in rack position 6. Select bake, set temperature 375 F, timer for 35 minutes. Press start to preheat the oven.
2. Add cracker crumbs and eggs in 2 separate shallow dishes.
3. Mix cracker crumbs with salt and pepper
4. Dip chicken in the eggs and then coat with cracker crumb.
5. Arrange coated chicken into the 9*13-inch baking dish.
6. Spread butter pieces on top of the chicken and bake for 30-35 minutes.

7. Serve and enjoy.

Nutrition: Calories 590, Fat 40, Carbs 9, Protein 46

Broccoli Bacon Ranch Chicken

Preparation Time: 15 minutes
Cooking Time: 30 minutes
Servings: 4
Ingredients:

- 4 chicken breasts, skinless and boneless
- 1/3 cup mozzarella cheese, shredded
- 1 cup cheddar cheese, shredded
- 1/2 cup ranch dressing
- 5 bacon slices, cooked and chopped
- 2 cups broccoli florets, blanched and chopped

Directions:

1. Insert wire rack in rack position 6. Select bake, set temperature 375 F, timer for 30 minutes. Press start to preheat the oven.
2. Add chicken into the 13*9-inch casserole dish. Top with bacon and broccoli.
3. Pour ranch dressing over chicken and top with shredded mozzarella cheese and cheddar cheese.
4. Bake chicken for 30 minutes.
5. Serve and enjoy.

Nutrition: Calories 551, Fat 30, Carbs 5, Protein 60

Jerk Chicken Legs

Preparation Time: 20 minutes
Cooking Time: 50 minutes
Servings: 10
Ingredients:

- 10 chicken legs
- 1/2 tsp. ground nutmeg
- 1/2 tsp. ground cinnamon
- 1 tsp. ground allspice

- 1 tsp. black pepper
- 1 tbsp. fresh thyme
- 1 1/2 tbsp. brown sugar
- 1/4 cup soy sauce
- 1/3 cup fresh lime juice
- 1 tbsp. ginger, sliced
- 2 habanera peppers, remove the stem
- 4 garlic cloves, peeled and smashed
- 6 green onions, chopped

Directions:

1. Add chicken into the large zip-lock bag.
2. Add remaining ingredients into the food processor and process until course. Pour mixture over chicken. Seal bag and shake well to coat the chicken and place it in the refrigerator overnight.
3. Insert wire rack in rack position 6. Select bake, set temperature 375 F, timer for 50 minutes. Press start to preheat the oven.
4. Line baking sheet with foil. Arrange marinated chicken legs on a baking sheet and bake for 45-50 minutes.
5. Serve and enjoy.

Nutrition: Calories 232, Fat 14, Carbs 5, Protein 21

Creamy Cheese Chicken

Preparation Time: 23 minutes
Cooking Time: 45 minutes
Servings: 4
Ingredients:

- 4 chicken breasts, skinless, boneless & cut into chunks
- 1 cup mayonnaise
- 1 tsp. garlic powder
- 1 cup parmesan cheese, shredded
- Pepper
- Salt

Directions:

1. Add chicken pieces into the bowl of buttermilk and soak overnight.
2. Insert wire rack in rack position 6. Select bake, set temperature 375 F, timer for 45 minutes. Press start to preheat the oven.
3. Add marinated chicken pieces into the 9*13-inch baking dish. Mix together mayonnaise, garlic powder, 1/2 cup parmesan cheese, pepper, and salt and pour over chicken.
4. Sprinkle remaining cheese on top of the chicken and bake for 40-45 minutes.
5. Serve and enjoy.

Nutrition: Calories 581; Fat 35, Carbs 15, Protein 50

Baked Chicken Breasts

Preparation Time: 13 minutes
Cooking Time: 20 minutes
Servings: 6
Ingredients:

- 6 chicken breasts, skinless & boneless
- 1/4 tsp. paprika
- 1/2 tsp. garlic salt
- 1 tsp. Italian seasoning
- 2 tbsp. olive oil
- 1/4 tsp. pepper

Directions:

1. Insert wire rack in rack position 6. Select bake, set temperature 390 F, timer for 25 minutes. Press start to preheat the oven.
2. Brush chicken with oil. Mix together Italian seasoning, garlic salt, paprika, and pepper and rub all over the chicken.
3. Arrange chicken breasts on a roasting pan and bake for 25 minutes or until internal temperature reaches 165 F.

4. Slice and serve.

Nutrition: Calories 321, Fat 15, Carbs 1, Protein 42

Flavors Balsamic Chicken

Preparation Time: 12 minutes
Cooking Time: 25 minutes
Servings: 4
Ingredients:

- 4 chicken breasts, skinless and boneless
- 2 tsp. dried oregano
- 2 garlic cloves, minced
- 1/2 cup balsamic vinegar
- 2 tbsp. soy sauce
- 1/4 cup of oil
- Pepper
- Salt

Directions:

1. Insert wire rack in rack position 6. Select bake, set temperature 390 F, timer for 25 minutes. Press start to preheat the oven.
2. In a bowl, mix together soy sauce, oil, black pepper, oregano, garlic, and vinegar.
3. Place chicken in a baking dish and pour soy sauce mixture over chicken. Let it sit for 10 minutes. Bake chicken for 25 minutes. Serve and enjoy.

Nutrition: Calories 401, Fat 23, Carbs 2, Protein 42

Simple & Delicious Chicken Thighs

Preparation Time: 10 minutes
Cooking Time: 35 minutes
Servings: 6
Ingredients:

- 6 chicken thighs
- 2 tsp. poultry seasoning

- 2 tbsp. oil
- Pepper
- Salt

Directions:

1. Insert wire rack in rack position 6. Select bake, set temperature 390 F, timer for 40 minutes. Press start to preheat the oven.
2. Brush chicken with oil and rub with poultry seasoning, pepper, and salt.
3. Arrange chicken on roasting pan and bake for 35-40 minutes or until internal temperature reaches 165 F.
4. Serve and enjoy.

Nutrition: Calories 319, Fat 15, Carbs 1, Protein 42

Perfect Baked Chicken Breasts

Preparation Time: 10 minutes
Cooking Time: 30 minutes
Servings: 4
Ingredients:

- 4 chicken breasts, bone-in & skin-on
- 1 tsp. oil (Olive)
- 1/4 tsp. black pepper
- 1/2 tsp. kosher salt

Directions:

1. Insert wire rack in rack position 6. Select bake, set temperature 375 F, timer for 30 minutes. Press start to preheat the oven.
2. Brush chicken with oil and season with salt
3. Place chicken on roasting pan and bake for 30 minutes.
4. Serve and enjoy.

Nutrition: Calories 288, Fat 12, Carbs 1, Protein 42

CHAPTER 10:

Optavia Vegan & Vegetarian

Vegan Pear and Cranberry Cake

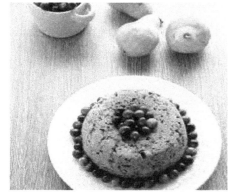

Preparation time: 5 minutes
Cooking Time: 45 minutes
Servings: 4-6
Ingredients:

- 1 1/4 cup whole wheat pastry flour
- 1/8 teaspoon sea salt
- baking powder
- baking soda
- 1/2 teaspoon ground cardamom
- Cup of halved unsweetened nondairy milk
- 2 tablespoons coconut oil
- 2 tablespoons ground flax seeds
- 1/4 cup agave
- 2 cups water
- Cup of halved chopped cranberries
- 1 cup chopped pear

Directions:

1. Grease a Bundt pan; set aside.

2. In a mixing, mix all dry ingredients together. In another bowl, mix all wet ingredients; whisk the wet ingredients into the dry until smooth.

3. Fold in the add-ins and spread the mixture into the pan; cover with foil.

4. Place pan in your air fryer toast oven and add water in the bottom and bake at 370 degrees F for 35 minutes.

5. When done, use a toothpick to check for doneness. If it comes out clean, then the cake is ready, if not, bake for 5-10 more minutes, checking frequently to avoid burning.

6. Remove the cake and let stand for 10 minutes before transferring from the pan. Enjoy!

Nutrition: Calories 309, Carbs 14, Fat 27, Protein 22

Oven Steamed Broccoli

Preparation time: 8 minutes
Cooking Time: 3 minutes
Servings: 2
Ingredients:

- 1 pound broccoli florets
- 1½ cups water
- Salt and pepper to taste
- I tsp. extra virgin olive oil

Directions:

1. Add water to the bottom of your air fryer toast oven and set the basket on top.

2. Toss the broccoli florets with salt pepper, and olive oil until evenly combined, then transfer to the basket of your air fryer toast oven.

3. Cook at 350 degrees for 5 minutes.

4. Remove the basket and serve the broccoli.

Nutrition: Calories 160, Fat 12, Carbs 6, Protein 13

Brussels sprouts

Preparation time: 11 minutes
Cooking Time: 13 minutes
Servings: 4
Ingredients:

- 2 pound Brussels sprouts, halved
- 1 tbsp. chopped almonds
- 1 tbsp. rice vinegar
- 2 tbsp. sriracha sauce
- 1/4 cup gluten-free soy sauce
- 2 tbsp. sesame oil
- 1/2 tbsp. cayenne pepper
- 1 tbsp. smoked paprika
- 1 tsp. onion powder
- 2 tsp. garlic powder
- 1 tsp. red pepper flakes
- Salt and pepper

Directions:

1. Preheat your air fryer toast oven to 370 degrees F.

2. Meanwhile, place your air fryer toast oven's pan on medium heat and cook the almonds for 3 minutes, then add in all the remaining ingredients.

3. Place the pan in the air fryer toast oven and cook for 8-10 minutes or until done to desire. Serve hot over a bed of steamed rice. Enjoy!

Nutrition: Calories 216, Fat 18, Carbs 9, Protein 18

Power Roasted Roots Soup

Preparation time: 18 minutes
Cooking Time: 1 hour
Servings: 5
Ingredients:

- 2 tablespoons extra virgin olive oil
- 2 red onions, quartered
- 2 red peppers, deseeded, chopped
- 3 tomatoes, halved
- 3 carrots, peeled, diced
- 2 sweet potatoes, peeled, diced
- 2 cans light coconut milk
- 1 teaspoon ground cumin
- 1 tablespoon smoked paprika, plus extra for garnish
- 2 inches fresh root ginger, peeled, minced
- 1 bay leaf
- Salt and black pepper
- Chopped coriander to garnish
- Lime wedges

Directions

1. Preheat oven your air fryer toast oven to 400°F.

2. In your air fryer toast oven's pan, mix all the veggies and oil and roast in the air fryer toast oven for about 40 minutes or until cooked.

3. Remove from air fryer toast oven.

4. Chop the roasted vegetables and place them in a saucepan; add the remaining ingredients and stir to mix well; season with salt and bring the mixture to a gentle boil in a saucepan and then simmer for about 20 minutes.

5. Divide the soup among six serving bowls and sprinkle each with coriander, black pepper, and smoked paprika.

6. Garnish with lime wedges and enjoy!

Nutrition: Calories 390, Carbs 11, Fat 22, Protein 19

Healthy Vegetable Sauté

Preparation time: 15 minutes
Cooking Time: **16 minutes**
Servings: 3
Ingredients:

- 2 tablespoons extra virgin olive oil
- 1 tablespoon minced garlic
- 1 large shallot, sliced
- 1 cup mushrooms, sliced
- 1 cup broccoli florets
- 1 cup artichoke hearts
- 1 bunch asparagus, sliced into 3-inch pieces
- 1 cup baby peas
- 1 cup cherry tomatoes, halved
- 1/2 teaspoon sea salt
- **Vinaigrette**
- 3 tablespoons white wine vinegar
- 6 tablespoons extra-virgin olive oil
- 1/2 teaspoon sea salt
- 1 teaspoon ground oregano
- Handful fresh parsley, chopped

Directions:

1. Add oil to the pan of your air fryer toast oven set over medium heat. Stir in garlic and shallots and sauté for about 2 minutes.
2. Stir in mushrooms for about 3 minutes or until golden.
3. Stir in broccoli, artichokes, and asparagus and continue cooking for 3 more minutes. Stir in peas, tomatoes, and salt and transfer to the air fryer toast oven and cook for 5-8 more minutes.
4. Prepare vinaigrette: mix together vinegar, oil, salt, oregano, and parsley in a bowl until well combined.
5. Serve vegetable sauté in a serving bowl and drizzle with vinaigrette.

6. Toss to combine and serve.

Nutrition: Calories 293, Fat 27, Carbs 14, Protein 25

Satisfying Grilled Mushrooms

Preparation time: 13 minutes
Cooking Time: 11 minutes
Servings: 4
Ingredients:

- 2 cups shiitake mushrooms
- 1 tablespoon balsamic vinegar
- 1/4 cup extra virgin olive oil
- 1-2 garlic cloves, minced
- A handful of parsley
- 1 teaspoon salt

Directions:

1. Rinse the mushroom and pat dry; put in a foil and drizzle with balsamic vinegar and extra virgin olive oil.
2. Sprinkle the mushroom with garlic, parsley, and salt.
3. Grill for about 10 minutes in your air fryer toast oven at 350 degrees F or until tender and cooked through.
4. Serve warm.

Nutrition: Calories 260, Fat 19, Carbs 11, Protein 22

Squash Pappardelle with Ricotta and Dried Tomato Sauce

Preparation time: 5 minutes
Cooking Time: 20 minutes
Servings: 4
Ingredients:

- 3 zucchini (ends trimmed)
- 3 medium squash (ends trimmed)
- 1 tsp. olive oil
- ½ tsp. salt
- Black pepper to taste

- ¼ cup sun-dried tomatoes (soaked in hot water for 10 minutes and drained)
- 1 tomato (seeded and coarsely chopped)
- 1 red bell pepper (halved and coarsely chopped)
- 1 garlic clove (minced)
- 1 tbsp. white balsamic vinegar
- 1 tbsp. olive oil
- ½ small shallot (diced)
- 12 fresh basil leaves (chopped)
- 1 cup ricotta cheese (part-skim)

Directions:

1. With a vegetable peeler, slice the zucchini and the squash lengthwise into paper-thin strips, then stack the strips and slice lengthwise to make ribbons (½ - inch thin).
2. Place the strips in a bowl and drizzle with oil, salt, black pepper, and sent them on the side to soften.
3. Meanwhile, put the drained sun-dried tomatoes in a food processor and blend for a few minutes to coarsely chop.
4. Add the fresh tomato, bell pepper, garlic, vinegar, and blend for a few minutes until just combined. While blending everything, slowly stream in oil, being careful not to over-process the mixture, since the sauce should be thick and a bit chunky.
5. Then, transfer to a bowl and fold in the red pepper flakes, shallot, and basil.
6. Serve.

Nutrition: Calories: 387 Fat: 6 g Carbohydrate: 14 gProtein: 18 g

Mini Pepper Nachos

Cooking time: 20 minutes
Preparation time: 20 minutes
Servings: 4 servings

Ingredients:

- ¼ cup jalapeño (diced)
- Cooking spray
- 1,12 oz. can chicken (in water) drained
- 6 oz. avocado (mashed)
- ½ cup Greek yogurt
- 2 cups shredded cheddar cheese (low-fat, divided)
- 1 tsp. chili powder
- 24 mini bell peppers (halved, remove stem, seeds, and membranes)
- ¼ cup scallions (chopped)

Directions:

1. In a lightly greased pan, sauté the jalapeño until tender.
2. In a bowl, mix the jalapeño, chicken, avocado, Greek yogurt, one cup of cheddar cheese, and chili powder.
3. Put the mini bell peppers in a single layer in a casserole dish. Fill with chicken mixture, sprinkle with the remaining cheese, and broil until cheese has melted (about 2-4 minutes).
4. Garnish with scallions and serve with salsa, if desired.

Nutrition: Calories: 132 Carbs: 21g Fat: 4g Protein: 3g

Yummy Baked Carrot Hummus

Preparation time: 15 minutes
Cooking Time: 25 minutes
Servings: 4
Ingredients:

- 1 pound carrots, peeled and chopped
- 19 ounces canned chickpeas, drained and rinsed
- 2 cloves garlic
- 4 tablespoons freshly squeezed lemon juice
- ½ teaspoon cumin
- 3 tablespoons tahini

- 2 ½ tablespoons olive oil
- Sea salt to taste

Directions

1. Toss the carrots and ½ a teaspoon olive oil in a roasting pan and bake up to 25 minutes at 400 degrees F in your air fryer toast oven.
2. Remove from oven and let cool slightly, then process in a blender or food processor with the remaining ingredients.
3. Enjoy!

Nutrition: Calories 181, Fat 16, Carbs 9, Protein 19

Warm Lemon Rosemary Olives

Preparation time: 15 minutes
Cooking Time: 20 minutes
Servings: 12
Ingredients

- 1 teaspoon extra-virgin olive oil
- 1 teaspoon grated lemon peel
- 1 teaspoon crushed red pepper flakes
- 2 sprigs fresh rosemary
- 3 cups mixed olives
- Lemon twists, optional

Directions:

1. Preheat your air fryer toast oven to 400 degrees F.
2. Place pepper flakes, rosemary, olives, and grated lemon peel onto a large sheet of foil; drizzle with oil and fold the foil.
3. Pinch the edges of the sheet to tightly seal.
4. Bake in the preheated air fryer toast oven for about 30 minutes.
5. Remove from the sheet and place the mixture in a serving dish.

6. Serve warm garnished with lemon twists.

Nutrition: Calories 146, Fat 14, Carbs 8, Protein 21

Cashews-and Pretzel-Crusted Tofu

Preparation time: 15 minutes
Cooking Time: 20 minutes
Servings: 4
Ingredients:

- 1 cup flour (Whole)
- 1 package (16-ounce) extra firm tofu, chopped into 8 slices
- ¾ cup raw cashews
- 2 cups pretzel sticks
- 1 tbsp. extra virgin olive oil
- 1 cup unsweetened almond milk
- 2 tsp. chili powder
- 2 tsp. garlic precipitate
- 2 tsp. onion powder
- 1 tsp. lemon pepper
- ¼ tsp. black pepper
- ½ tsp. sea salt

Directions:

1. Preheat your air fryer toast oven to 400 degrees F.
2. Line a baking sheet with baking paper and set aside.
3. In a food processor, pulse together cashews and pretzel sticks until coarsely ground.
4. Combine garlic, onion, chili powder, lemon pepper, and salt in a small bowl.
5. In a large bowl, combine half of the spice mixture and flour.
6. Add almond milk to a separate bowl.
7. In another bowl, combine cashew mixture, salt, pepper, and olive oil; mix well.
8. Sprinkle tofu slices with the remaining half of the spice mixture and coat each

with the flour and then dip in almond milk; coat with the cashew mixture and bake for about 18 minutes or until golden brown.

9. Serve the baked tofu with your favorite vegan salad.

Nutrition: Calories 332, Fat 8, Carbs 23, Protein 12

Kale Salad with Chickpeas and Spicy Tempeh Bits

Preparation time: 15 minutes
Cooking Time: 20 minutes
Servings: 4
Ingredients:
Tempeh Bits:

- ¼ cup vegetable oil
- 8 oz. tempeh
- 1 tsp. lemon pepper
- 1 tsp. chili powder
- 2 tsp. sweet paprika
- 2 tsp. garlic powder
- 2 tsp. onion powder
- ¼ tsp. sea salt
- ⅛ Tsp. cayenne pepper or more to taste

Salad:

- 15.5 oz. can chickpeas
- 1 lb. chopped kale
- 1 cup shredded carrots
- 2 tbsp. sesame seeds, toasted

Dressing:

- 1 tbsp. fresh grated ginger
- 2 tbsp. toasted sesame oil
- ¼ cup low sodium soy sauce
- ⅓ Cup seasoned rice vinegar

Directions:

1. Blanch kale in a pot of salted boiling water for about 30 seconds and immediately run under cold water; drain and squeeze out excess water. Set aside.

2. Preheat your air fryer toast oven to 425 degrees F.

3. In a small bowl, combine all the spices for tempeh.

4. Add oil to a separate bowl. Slice tempeh into thin pieces.

5. Dip each tempeh slice into the oil and arrange them on a paper-lined baking sheet; generously sprinkle with the spices until well covered and bake for about 20 minutes or until crispy and golden brown, then remove from air fryer toast oven. In a large bowl, combine all the salad ingredients and set aside.

6. In a jar, combine all the dressing ingredients; close and shake until well blended; pour the dressing over salad and toss to coat well.

7. Crumble the crispy tempeh on top of the salad to serve.

8. Enjoy!

Nutrition: Calories 308, Fat 7, Carbs 19, Protein 9.

Buffalo Cauliflower

Preparation time: 15 minutes
Cooking Time: 17 minutes
Servings: 4
Ingredients:

- 2 medium head Cauliflowers which should be carefully chopped to florets that can be eaten in one scoop
- 4-6 tablespoons of Red Hot Spice/Sauce. You can reduce this if you don't like spices a lot.
- ½ teaspoon of salt
- 2 tablespoon of arrowroot starch. You can also use cornstarch
- 3 teaspoons of maple syrup
- 4 spoons of your favorite avocado oil

- 4 tablespoons of nutritional yeast

Directions:

1. First of all, make sure to cook with your Air Fryer at 360F
2. Then add all your ingredients to a large bowl except the cauliflower.
3. Whisk the ingredients in the bowl until it is thorough.
4. Add the cauliflower and toss it to coat evenly.
5. Proceed to add half of your cauliflower to your new Air Fryer.
6. Cook for about 13 minutes, and you can shake halfway through the cooking process.
7. If you have leftovers, then you can reheat in your Air Fryer for about 2 minutes.

Nutrition: Calories 200, Fat 6, Carbs 20, Protein 8

Mozzarella Stalks

Preparation time: 20 minutes

Cooking Time: 30 minutes

Servings: 6

Ingredients:

- 15 Mozzarella sticks: cut from a block of cheese
- ½ cup general-purpose flour
- 2 Eggs
- 1½ cups Breadcrumbs
- Spices: onion powder, garlic powder, smoked paprika (1 tsp. each), and salt (to taste).
- Sauce: any of your choice

Directions:

1. Make your mozzarella sticks by cutting them straight from cheese blocks (you may have them pre-cut).
2. Arrange cheese sticks on a plate (parchment-lined for ease) and freeze in a freezer for about 40 minutes to

prevent melting when placed into the air fryer.

3. You may seize your flour to remove air bubbles and place it inside a covered bowl.
4. Break eggs into a bowl and whisk well.
5. Pour and mix spices and breadcrumb into a bowl.
6. Coat the mozzarella sticks evenly by placing them into the covered bowl or container, cover tightly, and shake. Open the bowl, take out the sticks one at a time, place them into the whisked egg, and then into the mixture of the spices and crumbs.
7. Place the coated sticks back on the plate and freeze for about 30 minutes more this time around.
8. Get your air fryer out and clean it (you can do that before the whole cooking process). Grease the air fryer racks lightly. Preheat the air fryer to 390°F.
9. Take out the mozzarella sticks from the freezer and once more, place them into the whisked egg, and then into the mixture of the spices and crumbs. Once you are done, transfer them to the air fryer in batches if they cannot all fit into the rack.
10. Set the timer to 7-10 minutes and cook until you have crispy, golden brown mozzarella sticks.
11. Serve with marinara or any sauce of your choice.

Nutrition: Calories 200, Fat 7, Carbs 120, Protein 9.

Vegan Fried Ravioli

Preparation time: 20 minutes

Cooking Time:

Servings: 2

Ingredients:

- ¼ Cup of Panko Bread crumbs
- ½ teaspoons of dried basil

- 1 teaspoon of your favorite nutritional yeast flakes
- Pinch of pepper and small salt to taste
- ¼ cup of aquafaba liquid from the can, or you can use other beans
- ½ teaspoon of garlic powder
- ½ teaspoon of dried oregano
- ¼ cup of marinara to dip
- 4 ounces of thawed vegan ravioli

Directions:

1. Combine the nutritional yeast flakes, dried oregano, salt, pepper, dried basil, garlic powder, and panko bread crumbs on a plate or a clean surface.
2. Put your aquafaba in a separate bowl
3. Carefully dip the ravioli in the aquafaba, and shake off the excess liquid.
4. After that, dredge it in the bread crumbs mixture while making sure that your ravioli is well covered.
5. Then, move the ravioli into the air fryer basket.
6. Do these steps for all the ravioli you want to cook.
7. Make sure to space the ravioli well in the air fryer basket to ensure that they can turn brown evenly
8. Then go on to spritz your ravioli with cooking spray in the air fryer basket
9. Set your air fryer to 390F
10. Cook for 7 minutes and carefully turn each ravioli on their sides. Try as much as possible not to shake the baskets as you will waste the bread crumbs. After turning, proceed to cook for 2 more minutes.
11. Your ravioli is ready to eat. Make sure to serve with warm marinara as a dipping.
12. Save your leftovers in the refrigerator and reheat when you are ready to eat.

Nutrition: Calories 308, Fat 4, Carbs 18, Protein 4.

Veg Pizza

Preparation time: 15 minutes
Cooking Time: 20 minutes
Servings: 4
Ingredients:

- Pizza
- Pizza sauce
- Olives (or other veg toppings of your choice)
- Cheese
- Basil
- Pepper flakes

Directions:

1. If you are just fetching the pizza out of the freezer, you might want to warm it. Set the air fryer to 350°F.
2. Once warm, top the pizza with the pizza sauce.
3. Add cheese to the pizza.
4. Add olives to the pizza.
5. Arrange the pizza carefully on the air fryer rack.
6. (NOTE: you can also set your dough into the air fryer rack before adding the toppings to prevent spills)
7. Preheat the air fryer to 350°F and spray the air fryer rack with oil. Set the timer to 5-7 minutes and cook until the cheese is melted.
8. Once cooked, let the cheese set on pizza by waiting for about 2-3 minutes before cutting. Serve warm while topping it with basil and pepper flakes.

Nutrition: Calories 280, Fat 10, Carbs 120, Protein 20.

Buffalo Cauliflower – Onion Dip

Preparation time:
Cooking Time:
Servings: 2
Ingredients:

- ¾ head of Cauliflower

- ¾ cup of Buffalo sauce
- Seasoning and spice: Garlic powder (1½ tsp.) and salt (to taste)
- Creamy dipping sauce: French onion dip (or any sauce of your choice)
- Celery
- 3 tbsp. Olive oil

Directions:

1. Cut the head of cauliflower into tiny florets into a big bowl.
2. Add and mix the cauliflower with the buffalo sauce and the rest of the ingredients apart from the dip sauce and celery sticks.
3. Grease the air fryer rack lightly. Preheat the air fryer to 375°F.
4. Transfer the well-mixed cauliflower to the air fryer in batches if they cannot all fit into the rack.
5. Set the timer to 10-12 minutes and cook until the cauliflower florets are tender and browned a bit.
6. Serve warm with the celery sticks and dipping sauce of your choice. In my own case, french onion dip.

Nutrition: Calories 200, Fat 4, Carbs 190, Protein 9.

Baked Apple

Preparation time: 15 minutes
Cooking Time: 25 minutes
Servings: 2
Ingredients:

- 2 Apples
- Oats (as a topping)
- 3 tsp. melted margarine/butter
- ½ tsp. Cinnamon
- ½ tsp. nutmeg powder
- 4 Tbsp. raisins
- ½ cup of water

Directions:

1. Wash and dry apples.
2. Cut the apples in half and use a spoon or knife to cut out some of the flesh.
3. Add the melted margarine, cinnamon, nutmeg powder, chopped raisins, and oats into a small bowl and mix.
4. Preheat the air fryer to 350°F.
5. Place the apples into the drip pan at the bottom of the air fryer.
6. Put the mixture into the center of the apples using a spoon.
7. Pour water into the pan.
8. Set the timer to 15-20 minutes for it to bake till apples are tender and fillings are crisp and browned.
9. Cover the fillings with foil if they seem to be browning quickly.
10. Serve warm and enjoy.

Nutrition: Calories 380, Fat 6, Carbs 170, Protein 14.

Eggplant Parmesan

Preparation time: 20 minutes
Cooking Time: 20 minutes
Servings: 3
Ingredients:

- 2 Eggplants
- 1 cup Whole wheat bread crumbs
- 1 cup Flour
- 1 cup Almond milk
- 4 tbsp. Vegan parmesan
- Spices: onion powder, pepper, garlic powder, and salt (to taste)
- Sauce: marinara
- Toppings: 1 cup mozzarella shreds

Directions:

1. Wash and dry eggplants.
2. Cut into slices.
3. Sieve flour to remove air bubbles into a bowl.

4. Mix whole wheat bread crumbs with vegan parmesan, onion powder, pepper, garlic powder, and salt together into a bowl.
5. Take the slices and dip into flour to be coated, then into the almond milk, and lastly into the mixture of vegan parmesan and spices.
6. Preheat the air fryer at 375°F.
7. Place eggplant slices into the air fryer rack.
8. Set the timer to 15-20 minutes, pressing the "Rotate" so that you can turn the slices halfway through.
9. Once golden brown on both sides, top with marinara and the mozzarella shreds and air fry for about 1-2 minutes to melt.
10. Serve warm and enjoy with pasta or any meal of your choice.

Nutrition: Calories 308, Fat 4, Carbs 54, Protein 8.

Vegan Cheese Samboosa

Preparation Time: 17 minutes
Cooking Time: 20 minutes
Serving: 3
Ingredients
For the Samboosa:

- ½ tablespoon of pure olive oil
- ¼ cup of water
- 1package of samoosa pastry sheet

For the Cheese:

- 1 ½ tablespoon of your favorite nutritional yeast
- ½ teaspoon of sea salt
- 1 ½ cup of water
- ¼ cup of raw cashew. It is best if you pre-boil for 9 minutes
- 2 ½ tablespoon and Tapioca starch (Don't use any other thickener apart

from Tapioca, it would yield undesirable results.)
- ½ teaspoon of Apple cider vinegar

Directions:

1. Use your blender to blend all the cheese ingredients using the "high" option until the mixture is smooth
2. Transfer the blended mixture into a saucepan, then heat at medium temperature. Use a spatula to stir while it cooks continuously.
3. Your mixture will turn into a big mass of cheese at about 4 minutes, and you will usually see the process start with the formation of clumps.
4. Cook for additional seconds to make sure it is well done.
5. Put it in the fridge to ensure that it cools before handling. This will take about 20 minutes.
6. After this, place a Samoosa pastry sheet on your cutting board and start adding water slightly using a clean pastry brush. This is to make sure that the edges will stick together.
7. Then, add about 1-2 teaspoons of the cheese mixture to the far right corner. Using the bottom right, carefully fold the pastry over the filling to form a triangular shape.
8. Take the top right point of the triangle and proceed to fold horizontally. You should do the previous two steps till you have a triangular shaped parcel, with the final flap sealed.
9. Repeat this till all your samoosa flaps are used.
10. Brush each samoosa with the pastry brush using the pure olive oil. Do this for each side.
11. Place 4-6 parcels of the Samoosa in your Air Fryer basket.
12. Cook at 385F for 7-9 minutes until it is crisp and well done.

13. Freeze the leftovers.

Nutrition: Calories 208, Fat 4, Carbs 190, Protein 19.

Delicious Potato Chips

Preparation time: 5 minutes

Cooking Time: 10 minutes

Servings: 4

Servings: 3

Ingredients:

- Grape seed oil cooking spray or any other cooking spray of your choice.

- Seasonings of choice.

- Pinch of sea salt according to your taste

- 2 medium-sized Russet Potato.

Directions:

1. Slice your potato after removing the outer cover. Make sure to slice into thin, cylindrical shapes. Use a paper towel to remove as much water from the thin potato slice. Don't do this too hard.

2. Use a teaspoon to add the seasoning of your choice uniformly to the potato slices. Then, spray your Air Fryer Basket with oil spray.

3. Place the sliced potatoes in a single layer inside the basket, you can do this in batches.

4. Go on to spray the top of the potato batches with grape seed oil spray and sprinkle with your sea salt.

5. Cook in your Air Fryer at 450F until the edges of the potatoes become golden brown. Depending on how thin your potato slices are, this should take about 15 minutes to cook in your Air Fryer.

6. Remove the crispy chips from your Fryer and let it cool down before eating.

7. You can store leftovers in the fridge.

Nutrition: Calories 160, Fat 6, Carbs 20, Protein 9.

CHAPTER 11:

Pork recipes

Pork Tenderloin

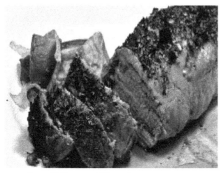

Preparation Time: 10 minutes
Cooking Time: 25 minutes
Servings: 4
Ingredients

- 1.5 lb. pork tenderloin
- 1 tbsp. olive oil
- 1/4 tsp. garlic powder
- 1/4 tsp. salt

Directions

1. Brine the tenderloin according to brining instructions, and this is optional. Take tenderloin out from the fridge 20 minutes before cooking. If it was brined, discard brine and rinse pork. Cut silver skin according to these given instructions.

2. Preheat air fryer toaster oven to 450F. In a bowl, mix olive oil, black pepper, and garlic powder. Add the salt If you did not brine the pork. Stir. Brush olive oil mixture all over tenderloin. Put tenderloin in the air fryer tray, bending it if needed for it to fit. Cook it for 10 minutes, or until it has reached the desired doneness as indicated on an instant-read thermometer, 145-160F has been recommended by the US Pork Board. This will take 8 to 15 extra minutes. Set aside for at least 5 minutes before slicing into 1/2 to 3/4 inch pieces. Serve immediately.

Nutrition: calories 321, fat 28, carbs 7, protein 42

Quick Pork Belly

Preparation Time: 20 minutes
Cooking Time: 65 minutes
Servings: 4
Ingredients

- 2 lb. piece of pork belly
- Olive oil spray
- Salt

Directions

1. Take out the pork belly, if you are using a packaged piece of pork belly, then there is no need to dry the skin.

2. Score the skin with a sharp knife by slicing the rind and taking care not to cut through to the meat underneath.

3. Put on the tray inside your air fryer toaster oven, rind side up. Spray equally with olive oil cooking spray.

4. Cover it equally and thickly with a layer of cracked salt. Set your air fryer toaster oven to 180C for 45 minutes, then check the pork belly, if you see one side cooking faster than the other, it can be a good idea to flip the rack 180 degrees.

5. Now turn the air fryer up to full (230C) and set more 15 minutes. Some pieces of pork will be ready after these steps, others might need more than 15 minutes. Your pork belly will be done when the crackling is hard and crispy.

6. Different air fryers can have their own cooking times, so be aware of this when making your pork belly. Some air fryers toaster oven may require more or less cooking time.

Nutrition: calories 390, fat 20, carbs 3, protein 34

Crispy Pork Cutlets

Preparation Time: 10 minutes
Cooking Time: 20 minutes
Servings: 4
Ingredients

- 1 lb. boneless pork chops
- 1/4 cup flour
- 1/4 tsp. pepper
- 1/2 tsp. salt
- 3/4 cup panko breadcrumbs
- 2 eggs
- 2 tbsp. mayonnaise
- 2 tsp. Dijon
- 1/2 tsp. apple cider vinegar
- 2 tsp. honey

Directions

1. Between the two layers on saran wrap, equally pound the pork chops until unless they are 1/4 inch thick. Put the flour, salt, and pepper to a plate and mix with a fork until well mixed. In a bowl, whisk the two eggs. On another plate, add the Panko breadcrumbs. Dip down each pork cutlet into the flour, shaking off any extra. Then dip down the floured pork into the egg wash. Now, dip the pork into the breadcrumbs. Press the meat into the breadcrumbs so there can be a good

coating. Arrange the cutlets in the Air fryer Toaster Oven and cook it at 390 degrees F for 10 to 12 minutes, or until unless the pork reaches an internal temperature of 165 degrees F. During cooking, prepare the honey Dijon dipping sauce, but mixing all of the ingredients together. Eat the cooked pork with the sauce.

Nutrition:
Calories: 190 Carbs: 33g Fat: 4g Protein: 6g

Panko Crusted Pork Chops

Preparation Time: 10 minutes
Cooking Time: 22 minutes
Servings: 2
Ingredients

- 1/4 tsp. salt
- 1/4 tsp. pepper
- 4 Boneless Pork chops
- 1 egg beaten
- 1 tbsp. Parmesan cheese
- 1 cup panko
- 1/2 tsp. granulated garlic
- 1/2 tsp. paprika
- 1/2 tsp. onion powder
- 1/2 tsp. chili powder

Directions

1. Preheat the air fryer toaster oven to 400 degrees while you prepare the pork chops. Spritz pork chops with salt on both sides and let it sit while you are preparing the seasonings and egg wash. Put the beaten egg in a bowl. Flip the pork chops over after 6 minutes if needed, spray with more olive oil spray and keep cooking for the remaining 6 minutes.

Nutrition: Calories: 220, Fat: 6, Protein: 27, Carbs: 13

Southern Style Pork Chops

Preparation Time: 10 minutes
Cooking Time: 25 minutes
Servings: 4
Ingredients

- 3 tbsp. buttermilk
- 4 pork chops
- Seasoning Salt to taste
- 1/4 cup flour
- Pork Seasoning
- 1 Ziploc bag
- Cooking oil spray
- Pepper to taste

Directions

1. Wash the pork chops and pat dry them. With the seasoning salt and pepper, season the pork chops. Pour the buttermilk over the pork chops. Put the pork chops in a Ziploc baggie with flour. Shake it to coat it completely. Marinate it for 30 minutes. Put the pork chops in the air fryer toaster oven. Spray the pork chops with cooking oil spray. Cook the pork chops at 380 degrees for 15 minutes. Turn the pork chops over to the other side after 10 minutes.

Nutrition: Calories: 173, Fat: 6, Protein: 22, Carbs: 7,

Damn Best Pork Chops

Preparation Time: 05 minutes
Cooking Time: 17 minutes
Servings: 2
Ingredients

- 2 Pork chops
- 1 1/2 tsp. salt
- 2 tbsp. brown sugar
- 1 tbsp. paprika
- 1 1/2 tsp. black pepper
- 2 tbsp. olive oil

- 1 tsp. ground mustard
- 1/2 tsp. onion powder
- 1/4 tsp. garlic powder

Directions

1. Preheat air fryer toaster oven to 400 degrees for 5 minutes. Wash pork chops with cool water and pat dry completely with a paper towel. In a bowl, add all the dry ingredients. Coat the pork chops with olive oil and brush in the mix. Brush it in well and liberally. Use all of the brushed mix for the 2 pork chops. Cook pork chops in air fryer toaster oven at 400 degrees for 12 minutes, turning pork chops over after 6 minutes if needed.

Nutrition: Calories: 198, Fat: 6g, Protein: 25g, Carbs: 10g, Fiber: 0g

Apple Stuffy Pork Chop

Preparation Time: 20 minutes
Cooking Time: 40 minutes
Servings: 4
Ingredients

- 4 Boneless Pork chops
- 2 tsp. salt
- 1/2 tsp. dried sage
- 1/4 tsp. nutmeg
- 1/2 tsp. garlic powder
- 1 apple sliced
- 1/4 tsp. cinnamon
- 1/4 tsp. paprika
- 1/4 tsp. ground nutmeg
- 1/2 onion
- 1/4 tsp. black pepper
- 1/2 tsp. dried sage
- 2 tsp. maple syrup
- 1/4 tsp. cinnamon
- 2 tsp. Dijon mustard
- 1/2 tbsp. light butter

- 1/4 cup celery chopped
- 1/2 tsp. garlic powder

Directions

1. Pound the pork to 3/4 inch thickness. In a bowl, mix Dijon mustard and maple syrup. Set it aside. Put remaining pork ingredients. Slice a deep pocket in pork chops, but careful not to cut all the way through. Brush spice mixture all over and inside pork chops. In a skillet, melt the butter on medium to high heat. Put apples, onion, Celery, and spiced for the apple stuffing. Mix it well. Cover it and cook for 8-10 minutes or until soft, stirring occasionally. Now fill each pocket with 1/4 of the stuffing mixture.

2. Preheat air fryer toaster oven to 400 degrees F. Spray basket with olive oil cooking spray. Put pork chops in a basket and air fry it for 3 minutes. Turn pork chops, brush with maple syrup/Dijon mixture, and air fry for about another 4 minutes if needed.

Nutrition: Calories: 378, Fat: 13, Protein: 33, Carbs: 8

Juicy Pork Chops

Preparation Time: 10 minutes
Cooking Time: 30 minutes
Servings: 3
Ingredients

- 3 Six ounce pork chops
- 2 tsp. olive oil
- Salt & pepper
- Garlic powder
- Smoked paprika

Directions

1. Coat the pork chops with olive oil but lightly. Season them with salt, pepper, garlic powder, and smoked paprika. Put in the Air Fryer toaster oven and cook at 380°F for 10-14 minutes,

turning the pork chops at the halfway cooking point if needed. Check it if cooked, and if not, then cook a little more if desired. Serve warm.

Nutrition: Calories: 287, Fat: 10g, Protein: 35, Carbs: 6,

Pork Chop with Brussels Sprout

Preparation Time: 20 minutes
Cooking Time: 35 minutes
Servings: 1
Ingredients

- 8 oz. pork chops
- 6 oz. Brussels sprouts
- Olive oil spray
- 1 tsp. olive oil
- 1/8 tsp. kosher salt
- 1 tsp. maple syrup
- 1/2 tsp. black pepper
- 1 tsp. Dijon mustard

Directions

1. Coat pork chop with olive oil cooking spray; sprinkle it with salt and 1/4 tsp. of the pepper. Mix together oil, syrup, mustard, and remaining 1/4 tsp. pepper in a bowl; add Brussels sprouts; coat it. Put pork chop on 1 side of the air fryer toaster oven tray and coated Brussels sprouts on the other side. Heat air fryer to 400°F, and cook until unless golden brown and pork is cooked to the required temperature.

Nutrition: calories: 337, Fat: 11, Protein: 40, Carbs: 21,

Pork Dumplings with Sauce

Preparation Time: 20 minutes
Cooking Time: 60 minutes
Servings: 6
Ingredients

- 4 cups chopped Bok Choy

- 2 tsp. Soy sauce
- 4 ounces ground pork
- 1 tsp. canola oil
- 1/4 tsp. red pepper
- Olive oil spray
- 18 dumpling wrappers
- 1 tbsp. garlic
- 1 tsp. toasted
- Sesame oil
- 1/2 tsp. brown sugar
- 1 tbsp. ginger
- 1 tbsp. chopped Scallions
- 2 tbsp. rice vinegar

Directions

1. Put canola oil in a skillet over medium to high heat. Put Bok Choy, and cook, mixing often, until unless wilted and mostly dry, 6 to 8 minutes. Put ginger and garlic; cook, mixing constantly, 1 minute. Shift Bok Choy mixture to a plate to cool it for 5 minutes. Pat down the mixture dry with a paper towel. Fold the wrapper over to make a half-moon shape, pressing corners to seal. Do the same with remaining wrappers and filling.
2. Coat the air fryer toaster oven tray with olive oil spray.
3. Put 6 dumplings in tray, leaving room between each; spray the dumplings with olive oil spray.

Nutrition: Calories: 140, Fat: 5, Protein: 7, Carbs: 16,

Mozzarella Pork Belly Cheese
Preparation Time: 10 minutes
Cooking Time: 35 minutes
Servings: 4
Ingredients

- 3 tsp. olive oil
- 8 basil leaves

- 8 oz. Pork Belly
- 2 tomatoes
- 1/2 tsp. dried thyme
- 1/2 tsp. salt
- 1 tsp. dried oregano
- 1 tsp. dried basil
- 1/2 tsp. black pepper
- 4 oz. mozzarella cheese

Directions

1. Dry pork belly using the paper towels and discard the paper towels. Brush olive oil over the pork belly. Put seasonings, and mix pork belly to coat all of it with seasonings. Now open pork belly, line 4 pieces, and top with about 4 slices of tomatoes and 4 basil leaves. Close down the pork belly and seal it with 4 toothpicks at the corners of the pork belly. Do the same with another pork belly. Spritz Air Fryer basket with olive oil cooking spray. Lay the pork belly. Spray the top of the pork belly with olive oil cooking spray for a golden color. Set down the temperature to 360 degrees F and the set timer for 28 minutes or a bit more for desired crispness and golden brown color. When time completes, remove pork belly from baskets, and take out the toothpicks before serving. Garnish them with chopped basil.

Nutrition: Calories: 267, Fat: 20g, Protein: 12g, Carbs: 5g, Fiber: 0.5g

Zucchini Lean Pork Burger
Preparation Time: 20 minutes
Cooking Time: 25 minutes
Servings: 5
Ingredients

- 6 oz. zucchini
- Oil spray
- 1/4 cup breadcrumbs

- 1 clove garlic
- 1 tbsp. red onion
- 1 lb. lean pork
- 1 tsp. kosher salt, pepper

Directions

1. Squeeze all the moisture very well from the zucchini with paper towels. In a bowl, mix the ground pork, zucchini, breadcrumbs, garlic, onion, salt, and pepper. Create 5 equal patties, 4 oz. each, 1/2 inch thick. Preheat the air fryer toaster oven to 370F. Now cook in a single layer in two batches for 10 minutes or cook until browned and cooked through from the center.

Nutrition: Calories: 212, Fat: 14, Protein: 15, Carbs: 5,

Roasted Pepper Pork Prosciutto

Preparation Time: 20 minutes
Cooking Time: 60 minutes
Servings: 8
Ingredients

- 24 oz. pork cutlets
- Olive oil spray
- 12 oz. slices thin prosciutto
- 4 slices mozzarella
- 22 oz. roasted peppers
- 1 lemon
- 24 Spinach leaves
- 1 tbsp. olive oil
- 1/2 cup GF breadcrumbs
- Salt and fresh pepper

Directions

1. First, wash and dry the pork cutlets very well with paper towels. Add breadcrumbs to a bowl and in another second bowl, stir the olive oil, lemon juice, and pepper. Preheat the air fryer toaster oven to 450°F. Slightly spray a baking dish with olive oil spray. Put each cutlet on a work surface such as a cutting board and lay 1/2 slice prosciutto, 1/2 slice cheese, 1 piece of roasted pepper, and 3 spinach leaves on one side of the pork cutlet. Roll it and put the seam side down on a dish. Dip down the pork in the olive oil and lemon juice after that into the breadcrumbs. Do the same with the pork left. Bake it for 25 to 30 minutes or until your desired crispness.

Nutrition: Calories: 268, Fat: 16g, Protein: 24g, Carbs: 7g, Fiber: 1g

Creamy Pork Belly Rolls

Preparation Time: 20 minutes
Cooking Time: 55 minutes
Servings: 8
Ingredients

- 16 oz. Pork Belly
- Olive oil spray
- 2 oz. cream cheese
- 1/2 cup hot sauce
- 1/3 cup shredded carrots
- 1/2 cup blue cheese
- 1/3 cup chopped Scallions
- 16 egg roll wrappers

Directions

1. Add pork belly to the slow cooker and put enough water or pork broth to cover it well. Cook it high for 4 hours. Take it out and shred with two forks, remove the liquid. To prepare in the Instant Pot, put at least 1 cup broth or water, enough to cover the pork well. Cook it on high pressure for 15 minutes on natural release. Remove liquid and shred it with two forks. During the time, add the cream cheese and hot sauce together until it is smooth. Put the pork, blue cheese, carrots and scallions and stir well, makes 3 cups. Place egg roll wrapper at

a time on a clean surface, points facing top and bottom like a diamond. Spread 3 tbsp. of the buffalo dip mixture onto the bottom third of the wrapper. Dip down your finger in a bowl of water and rub it along the edges of the wrapper. Lift the nearest point to you and wrap it around the filling. Wrap the left and right corners toward the center and continue to roll into air-tight cylinder. Left aside and do the same with remaining wrappers and filling. Spray all sides of the egg rolls with olive oil spray using your fingers to equally coat. Preheat the air fryer toaster oven to 400F. Spritz a sheet pan with oil. Shift the egg rolls to the baking sheet and cook until unless browned and crisp, about 16 to 18 minutes, flipping halfway if needed. Eat immediately, with dipping sauce on the side, if needed. You can cook it more for the desired crispness.

Nutrition: Calories: 305, Fat: 16, Protein: 16, Carbs: 24,

Seasoned Bleu Pork Belly
Preparation Time: 15 minutes
Cooking Time: 35 minutes
Servings: 6
Ingredients:

- 36 oz. Pork belly
- 1/2 cup seasoned breadcrumb
- 2 large egg whites
- 1 large egg - Salt and pepper
- Cooking spray
- 4.4 oz. cheese

Direction

1. Preheat air fryer toaster oven to 450°F. Spray a large baking sheet with cooking spray. Wash down and dry the pork cutlets; lightly pound the pork to make thinner and lightly season with salt and pepper. Put pork onto the baking sheet

seems side down. Spray the top of the pork with more olive oil spray and bake it for about 25 minutes, or until your desired crispness and golden brownish color.

Nutrition: calories: 356, Fat: 20, Protein: 27, Carbs: 8,

Easy Cook Pork
Preparation Time: 15 minutes
Cooking Time: 45 minutes
Servings: 4
Ingredients: ¼ tsp. garlic powder

- 1/2 tsp. salt
- 1/4 tsp. smoked paprika
- 2 tbsp. butter
- 1/4 tsp. black pepper
- 4 boneless skinless Pork

Directions

1. In a bowl, mix butter, salt, garlic powder, smoked paprika, and pepper. Rub both sides of pork with butter mixture. Put the pork in air fryer toaster oven tray, standing against sides of the basket if needed. Set it to 350°F; cook it for 15 minutes or until juice of pork is clear when the center of thickest part is cut (at least 165°F). You can cook it a little bit more for the desired crispness.

Nutrition: Calories: 362, Fat: 21, Protein: 30, Carbs: 4

No Bread Pork Belly
Preparation Time: 15 minutes
Cooking Time: 95 minutes
Servings: 4
Ingredients:

- Kosher salt
- Olive oil spray
- 12 oz. Pork belly
- 1/2 tsp. parsley

- 3/4 tsp. garlic powder
- 1/8 cayenne pepper
- 3/4 tsp. onion powder
- 1/2 tsp. paprika

Directions

1. Slice the pork belly to even pieces.
2. Fill a bowl with 6 cups of light warm water and include 1/4 cup kosher salt, mix to dissolve.
3. Put the pork belly in the water and let them sit, refrigerate it for at least 1 to 1 1/2 hours to brine. Take it out from the water, pat dry with paper towels, and remove the water.
4. In a bowl, add 3/4 tsp. salt, with the left spices. Spray the pork with oil and rub all over, then rub the spice mix over the pork. Preheat the air fryer toaster oven to 350 degrees F.
5. Now heat an oven-safe or cast-iron skillet over high heat for 5 minutes until it becomes hot. Put the pork on the hot skillet, and cook it for 1 more minute. Rotate, and cook 1 minute from the other side. Shift skillet to the oven and bake it until unless no longer pink in the center and the juices run clear, and a thermometer reads 165 degrees F inserted in the center, about 8 to 10 minutes. You can cook it a little bit more for the desired crispness.

Nutrition: Calories: 258, Fat: 14, Protein: 29, Carbs: 5

Rustic Pork Ribs

Preparation Time: 5 minutes
Cooking Time: 25 minutes
Servings: 4
Ingredients:

- 1 rack of pork ribs
- 3 tablespoons dry red wine
- 1 tablespoon soy sauce
- 1/2 teaspoon dried thyme
- 1/2 teaspoon onion powder
- 1/2 teaspoon garlic powder
- 1/2 teaspoon ground black pepper
- 1 teaspoon smoke salt
- 1 tablespoon cornstarch
- 1/2 teaspoon olive oil

Directions:

1. Begin by preheating your air fryer oven to 390 degrees F. Place all ingredients in a mixing bowl and let them marinate for at least 1 hour.
2. Pour into the Oven rack/basket. Place the Rack on the middle-shelf of the Air fryer oven. Set temperature to 390°F, and set time to 25 minutes. Cook the marinated ribs for approximately 25 minutes.
3. Serve hot.

Nutrition: Calories: 268, Fat: 16, Protein: 24, Carbs: 7

CHAPTER 12:

Optavia Snack Recipes

Roasted Zucchini Boats with Ground Beef

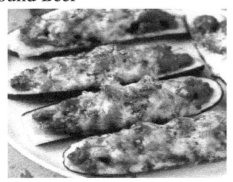

Preparation Time: 15 minutes
Cooking Time: 35 minutes
Servings: 8
Ingredients:

- Cooking spray
- 4 medium zucchinis
- 1 tablespoon olive oil
- 4 ounces cremini mushrooms, diced
- 2 garlic cloves, minced
- 8 ounces 90% lean ground beef
- ½ cup jarred tomato sauce
- ¼ teaspoon salt
- ⅛ teaspoon freshly ground black pepper
- ½ cup shredded part-skim mozzarella cheese

Directions:

1. Preheat the oven to 350°F. Coat a baking dish with cooking spray. Halve the zucchini lengthwise and, using a teaspoon, scoop out the seeds. Place the zucchini in the baking pan, leaving space between each zucchini.

2. In a large sauté pan or skillet over medium heat, heat the olive oil. Add the mushrooms and sauté until softened. Mix in garlic and cook until translucent. Add the ground beef and cook for 5 minutes, until browned, breaking up the pieces. Add the tomato sauce, salt, and pepper, and stir to combine. Continue until totally cooked. Let it cool for about 10 minutes.

3. Spoon 2 heaping tablespoons of beef mixture into each zucchini boat, and top each boat with 1 tablespoon of shredded mozzarella. Bake until it's cook.

Nutrition: calories 197, fat 5, carbs 4, protein 9

Spiced Popcorn
Preparation Time: 5 minutes
Cooking Time: 5 minutes
Servings: 4
Ingredients:

- 3 tablespoons olive oil
- ½ cup popcorn kernels
- Cooking spray
- 1 teaspoon garlic powder
- 1 teaspoon onion powder
- ½ teaspoon smoked paprika
- ½ teaspoon salt
- ⅛ teaspoon cayenne pepper

Directions:

1. Heat the olive oil in the pot. Add 3 popcorn kernels, and when one of the kernels pops, add the rest. Cover and shake well until fully popped, transfer the popcorn to a large bowl.

2. Spray the popcorn with cooking spray. Use clean hands to toss the popcorn, mixing it thoroughly. In a small bowl, mix together the garlic powder, onion powder, paprika, salt, and cayenne. Add some spice mix of your taste and toss until coated.

Nutrition: calories 210, fat 17, carbs 3, protein 16

Baked Spinach Chips

Preparation Time: 5 minutes
Cooking Time: 15 minutes
Servings: 4
Ingredients:

- Cooking spray
- 5 ounces baby spinach, washed and patted dry
- 2 tablespoons olive oil
- 1 teaspoon garlic powder
- ½ teaspoon salt
- ⅛ teaspoon freshly ground black pepper

Directions:

1. Preheat the oven to 350°F. Coat two baking sheets with cooking spray. Place the spinach in a large bowl. Mix in olive oil, garlic powder, salt, and pepper, and toss until evenly coated.

2. Spread the spinach in a single layer on the baking sheets. Bake until the spinach leaves are crispy and slightly browned. Store spinach chips in a resealable container at room temperature for up to 1 week.

Nutrition: calories 451, fat 18, carbs 7, protein 12

Peanut Butter Yogurt Dip with Fruit

Preparation Time: 10 minutes
Cooking Time: 5 minutes
Servings: 4
Ingredients:

- 1 cup nonfat vanilla Greek yogurt
- 2 tablespoons natural creamy peanut butter - 2 teaspoons honey
- 1 pear, cored and sliced
- 1 apple, cored and sliced
- 1 banana, sliced

Directions:

1. Whisk together the yogurt, peanut butter, and honey in a bowl. Serve the dip with the fruit on the side.

Nutrition: calories 421, fat 5, carbs 3, protein 10

Snickerdoodle Pecans

Preparation Time: 10 minutes
Cooking Time: 15 minutes
Servings: 8
Ingredients: Cooking spray

- 1½ cups raw pecans
- 2 tablespoons brown sugar
- 2 tablespoons 100% maple syrup
- ½ teaspoon ground cinnamon
- ½ teaspoon vanilla extract
- ⅛ teaspoon salt

Directions:

1. Line and set the oven to 350°F. spray. In a medium bowl, place the pecans. Add the brown sugar, maple syrup, cinnamon, vanilla, and salt, tossing to evenly coat.

2. Place pecans in a single layer. Bake for about 12 minutes, until pecans are lightly browned and fragrant. Remove and let it cool for 10 minutes.

Nutrition: calories 321, fat 28, carbs 7, protein 42

Almond-Stuffed Dates

Preparation Time: 5 minutes

Cooking Time: 3 minutes

Servings: 4

Ingredients:

- 20 raw almonds
- 20 pitted dates

Directions:

1. Stuffed one almond into each of 20 dates. Serve at room temperature.

Nutrition: calories 223, fat 12, carbs 4, protein 12

Peanut Butter Chocolate Chip Energy Bites

Preparation Time: 35 minutes

Cooking Time: 5 minutes

Servings: 12

Ingredients:

- 1 cup gluten-free old-fashioned oats
- ¾ cup natural creamy peanut butter
- ½ cup unsweetened coconut flakes
- ½ teaspoon vanilla extract
- 2 tablespoons honey
- ¼ cup dark chocolate chips

Directions:

1. Line the sheet and preheat the oven to 350°F. Spread the oats. Bake until the oats are browned. Let it cool.
2. Blend the oats, peanut butter, coconut, vanilla, and honey until smooth. Transfer the batter into a medium bowl, and fold in the chocolate chips. Spoon out a tablespoon of batter. Use clean hands to roll into a 2-inch ball and place on the baking sheet. Repeat for the remaining batter, making a total of 12 balls. Let it chill to set.

Nutrition: calories 333, fat 18, carbs 7, protein 12

No-Cook Pistachio-Cranberry Quinoa Bites

Preparation Time: 30 minutes

Cooking Time: 0 minutes

Servings: 12

Ingredients

- ½ cup quinoa
- ¾ cup natural almond butter
- ¾ cup gluten-free old-fashioned oats
- 2 tablespoons honey
- ⅛ teaspoon salt
- ¼ cup unsalted shelled pistachios, roughly chopped
- ¼ cup dried cranberries

Directions:

1. Blend the quinoa and blend until it turns into a flour consistency. Mix in almond butter, oats, honey, and salt, and blend until smooth.
2. Transfer into a medium bowl, and gently fold in the pistachios and cranberries. Spoon out a tablespoon of the batter. Use clean hands to roll into a 2-inch ball and place into a container. Repeat for the remaining batter, making a total of 12 balls. Let it chill to set.

Nutrition: calories 214, fat 19, carbs 3, protein 21

No-Bake Honey-Almond Granola Bars

Preparation Time: 15 minutes, plus 1 to 2 hours to chill

Cooking Time: 0 minutes

Servings: 8

Ingredients:

- Cooking spray - 1 cup pitted dates
- ¼ cup honey
- ¾ cup natural creamy almond butter
- ¾ cup gluten-free rolled oats

- 2 tablespoons raw almonds, chopped
- 2 tablespoons pumpkin seeds

Directions:

1. Line an 8-by-8-inch baking dish with parchment paper, and coat the paper with cooking spray. In a food processor or blender, add the dates and blend until they reach a paste-like consistency. Add the honey, almond butter, and oats, and blend until well combined. Transfer the mixture to a medium bowl.

2. Mix almonds and pumpkin seeds, and gently fold until well combined. Spoon the mixture into the prepared baking dish. Spread the mixture evenly, using clean fingers to push down the mixture, so it is compact. Let it chill for at least 1 to 2 hours. Remove from the refrigerator and cut into 8 bars. Carefully remove each bar from the baking dish, and wrap individually in plastic wrap. Place bars in the refrigerator until ready to grab and go.

Nutrition: calories 121, fat 1, carbs 8, protein 12

Cottage Cheese-Filled Avocado

Preparation Time: 5 minutes
Cooking Time: 3 minutes
Servings: 4
Ingredients:

- ½ cup low-fat cottage cheese
- ¼ cup cherry tomatoes, quartered
- 2 avocados, halved and pitted
- 4 teaspoons pumpkin seeds
- ¼ teaspoon salt
- ⅛ teaspoon freshly ground black pepper

Directions:

1. Mix together the cottage cheese and tomatoes in a bowl. Spoon 2 tablespoons of the cheese-tomato mixture onto each of the avocado halves. Top each with 1 teaspoon of pumpkin seeds, and sprinkle with salt and pepper.

Nutrition: calories 212, fat 15, carbs 3, protein 18

Toast with Balsamic Glaze

Preparation Time: 5 minutes
Cooking Time: 10 minutes
Servings: 2
Ingredients:

- 1 tablespoon brown sugar
- 5 cherry tomatoes, halved
- ⅛ teaspoon salt
- ⅛ teaspoon freshly ground black pepper

Directions:

1. Mix vinegar and brown sugar in a hot saucepan, continue stirring until it dissolves. Bring the mixture and simmer until the vinegar is reduced by half and thickens. Let it cool for 10 minutes.

2. Take out the flesh and mash it into the toasted bread. Topped it with tomatoes and seasoned. Then add the balsamic glaze to each toast.

Nutrition: calories 214, fat 8, carbs 4, protein 10

Whole-Wheat Chocolate-Banana Quesadillas

Preparation Time: 5 minutes
Cooking Time: 5 minutes
Servings: 4
Ingredients: Cooking spray

- 2 (10-inch) whole-wheat tortillas
- 1½ ounces 60% dark chocolate
- 2 tablespoons natural creamy peanut butter
- 1 medium banana, thinly sliced

Directions:

1. Add a tortilla and warm for 30 seconds on each side in a pan. Melt the chocolate in the microwave, about 1 minute, stirring halfway through. Using a spatula, spread the peanut butter onto 1 tortilla to the edges. Top with the banana slices, and drizzle the chocolate over the peanut butter.

2. Topped with the second tortilla, pressing down gently with the palm of your hand. Cut into 8 pieces and serve.

Nutrition: calories 212, fat 5, carbs 3, protein 10

Whole-Grain Mexican-Style Rollups

Preparation Time: 3 hours and 10 minutes

Cooking Time: 3 minutes

Servings: 4

Ingredients: ½ cup nonfat plain Greek yogurt

- ½ cup reduced-fat sour cream
- ¼ teaspoon salt
- 1⅛ teaspoon freshly ground black pepper
- 1 cup shredded pepper Jack cheese
- 1 15oz can low-sodium black beans
- 2 10-inch whole-wheat tortillas

Directions:

1. Mix together the yogurt, sour cream, salt, and pepper. Stir in the cheese and mashed beans. Lay the tortillas side by side on a cutting board. Spread 1 cup of the mixture onto each tortilla out to the edges.

2. Roll up each tortilla and cut off the uneven ends. Wrap each in plastic wrap and refrigerate for 1 to 2 hours. Cut each into 1-inch rollups.

Nutrition: calories 309, fat 8, carbs 4, protein 10

Chicken Nacho Bites

Preparation Time: 15 minutes

Cooking Time: 10 minutes

Servings: 4

Ingredients:

- Cooking spray
- ¾ cup low-sodium black beans, drained and rinsed
- ½ teaspoon hot sauce
- ¼ teaspoon salt
- 20 corn tortilla chips
- 3 ounces rotisserie chicken, coarsely chopped into 20 bite-size pieces
- ½ cup shredded reduced-fat sharp Cheddar cheese

Directions:

1. Preheat the oven to 400°F. Coat two baking sheets with cooking spray. Mix and toss beans, hot sauce, and salt. Mash until coarse.

2. Place tortilla chips. Topped the chip with black bean mixture, 1 piece of chicken, and 1 teaspoon of cheese. Bake until the cheese has melted.

Nutrition: calories 290, fat 1, carbs 3, protein 19

Snack Pizza with Chicken and Mushrooms

Preparation Time: 10 minutes

Cooking Time: 10 minutes

Servings: 4

Ingredients:

- Cooking spray
- 6 button mushrooms, chopped
- 3 ounces leftover chicken, chopped into bite-size pieces
- 4 whole-wheat English muffins
- 1 cup jarred tomato sauce
- ½ cup shredded part-skim mozzarella cheese

Directions:

1. Preheat the oven to 350°F. Coat with cooking spray. Mix together the mushrooms and chicken. Split each of the English muffins and place crust-side down on the prepared baking sheet, leaving about 1 inch between them. Top each with 2 tablespoons of tomato sauce, and spread the sauce to the bread. Top the tomato sauce with 3 tablespoons of the mushroom-chicken mixture, then 1 tablespoon of cheese.
2. Bake until cheese has melted and the bread is slightly toasted. Remove and let it cool for 10 minutes before serving.

Nutrition: calories 219, fat 12, carbs 2, protein 5

Crab Dip

Preparation time: *10 minutes*
Cooking time: *1 hour*
Servings: *2*
Ingredients:

- 2 ounces crabmeat
- 1 tablespoon lime zest, grated
- ½ tablespoon lime juice
- 2 tablespoons mayonnaise
- 2 green onions, chopped
- 2 ounces cream cheese, cubed
- Cooking spray

Directions:

1. Grease your slow cooker with the cooking spray, and mix the crabmeat with the lime zest, juice, and the other ingredients inside.
2. Put the lid on, cook on Low for 1 hour, divide into bowls, and serve as a party dip.

Nutrition: calories 209, fat 2, carbs 7, protein 14

Lemony Shrimp Dip

Preparation time: *10 minutes*
Cooking time: *2 hours*
Servings: *2*
Ingredients:

- 3 ounces cream cheese, soft
- ½ cup heavy cream
- 1 pound shrimp, peeled, deveined, and chopped
- ½ tablespoon balsamic vinegar
- 2 tablespoons mayonnaise
- ½ tablespoon lemon juice
- A pinch of salt and black pepper
- 2 ounces mozzarella, shredded
- 1 tablespoon parsley, chopped

Directions:

1. In your slow cooker, mix the cream cheese with the shrimp, heavy cream, and the other ingredients, whisk, put the lid on and cook on Low for 2 hours.
2. Divide into bowls and serve as a dip.

Squash Salsa

Preparation time: *10 minutes*
Cooking time: *3 hours*
Servings: *2*
Ingredients:

- 1 cup butternut squash, peeled and cubed
- 1 cup cherry tomatoes, cubed
- 1 cup avocado, peeled, pitted, and cubed
- ½ tablespoon balsamic vinegar
- ½ tablespoon lemon juice
- 1 tablespoon lemon zest, grated
- ¼ cup veggie stock
- 1 tablespoon chives, chopped
- A pinch of rosemary, dried
- A pinch of sage, dried

- A pinch of salt and black pepper

Directions:

1. In your slow cooker, mix the squash with the tomatoes, avocado, and the other ingredients, toss, put the lid on and cook on Low for 3 hours.
2. Divide into bowls and serve as a snack.

Nutrition: calories 3886, fat 6, carbs 4, protein 12

Flavory Beans Spread

Preparation time: *10 minutes*
Cooking time: *6 hours*
Servings: *2*
Ingredients: 1 cup canned black beans, drained - 2 tablespoons tahini paste

- ½ teaspoon balsamic vinegar
- ¼ cup veggie stock
- ½ tablespoon olive oil

Directions:

1. In your slow cooker, mix the beans with the tahini paste and the other ingredients, toss, put the lid on and cook on Low for 6 hours.
2. Transfer to your food processor, blend well, divide into bowls, and serve.

Nutrition: calories 432, fat 12, carbs 6, protein 4

Rice Bowls

Preparation time: *10 minutes*
Cooking time: *6 hours*
Servings: *2*
Ingredients:

- ½ cup wild rice
- 1 red onion, sliced
- ½ cup brown rice
- 2 cups veggie stock
- ½ cup baby spinach
- ½ cup cherry tomatoes, halved
- 2 tablespoons pine nuts, toasted
- 1 tablespoon raisins

- 1 tablespoon chives, chopped
- 1 tablespoon dill, chopped
- ½ tablespoon olive oil
- A pinch of salt and black pepper

Directions:

1. In your slow cooker, mix the rice with the onion, stock, and the other ingredients, toss, put the lid on, and cook on Low for 6 hours.
2. Divide into bowls and serve as a snack.

Nutrition: calories 211, fat 3, carbs 3, protein 10

Cauliflower Spread

Preparation time: *10 minutes*
Cooking time: *7 hours*
Servings: *2*
Ingredients: 1 cup cauliflower florets

- 1 tablespoon mayonnaise
- ½ cup heavy cream
- 1 tablespoon lemon juice
- ½ teaspoon garlic powder
- ¼ teaspoon smoked paprika
- ¼ teaspoon mustard powder
- A pinch of salt and black pepper

Directions:

1. In your slow cooker, combine the cauliflower with the cream, mayonnaise, and the other ingredients, toss, put the lid on and cook on Low for 7 hours.
2. Transfer to a blender, pulse well, into bowls, and serve as a spread.

Flavory Mushroom Dip

Preparation time: *10 minutes*
Cooking time: *5 hours*
Servings: *2*
Ingredients:

- 4 ounces white mushrooms, chopped

- 1 eggplant, cubed
- ½ cup heavy cream
- ½ tablespoon tahini paste
- 2 garlic cloves, minced
- A pinch of salt and black pepper
- 1 tablespoon balsamic vinegar
- ½ tablespoon basil, chopped
- ½ tablespoon oregano, chopped

Directions:

1. In your slow cooker, mix the mushrooms with the eggplant, cream, and the other ingredients, toss, put the lid on and cook on High for 5 hours.
2. Divide the mushroom mix into bowls and serve as a dip.

Nutrition: calories 189, fat 3, carbs 4, protein 3

Chickpeas Spread

Preparation time: *10 minutes*
Cooking time: *8 hours*
Servings: *2*
Ingredients: ½ cup chickpeas, dried

- 1 tablespoon olive oil
- 1 tablespoon lemon juice
- 1 cup veggie stock
- 1 tablespoon tahini
- A pinch of salt and black pepper
- 1 garlic clove, minced
- ½ tablespoon chives, chopped

Directions:

1. In your slow cooker, combine the chickpeas with the stock, salt, pepper, and garlic, stir, put the lid on and cook on Low for 8 hours.
2. Drain chickpeas, transfer them to a blender, add the rest of the ingredients, pulse well, divide into bowls and serve as a party spread.

Nutrition: calories 109, fat 2, carbs 2, protein 12

Spinach Dip

Preparation time: *10 minutes*
Cooking time: *1 hour*
Servings: *2*
Ingredients:

- 2 tablespoons heavy cream
- ½ cup Greek yogurt
- ½ pound baby spinach
- 2 garlic cloves, minced
- Salt and black pepper to the taste

Directions:

1. In your slow cooker, mix the spinach with the cream and the other ingredients, toss, put the lid on and cook on High for 1 hour.
2. Blend using an immersion blender, divide into bowls and serve as a party dip.

Nutrition: calories 221, fat 2, carbs 1, protein 3

Potato Salad

Preparation time: *10 minutes*
Cooking time: *8 hours*
Servings: *2*
Ingredients:

- 1 red onion, sliced
- 1 pound gold potatoes, peeled and roughly cubed
- 2 tablespoons balsamic vinegar
- ½ cup heavy cream
- 1 tablespoons mustard
- A pinch of salt and black pepper
- 1 tablespoon dill, chopped
- ½ cup celery, chopped

Directions:

1. In your slow cooker, mix the potatoes with the cream, mustard, and the other ingredients, toss, put the lid on and cook on Low for 8 hours.

2. Divide salad into bowls, and serve as an appetizer.

Nutrition: calories 218, fat 8, carbs 2, protein 4

Stuffed Peppers

Preparation time: *10 minutes*

Cooking time: *4 hours*

Servings: *2*

Ingredients:

- 1 red onion, chopped
- 1 teaspoons olive oil
- ½ teaspoon sweet paprika
- ½ tablespoon chili powder
- 1 garlic clove, minced
- 1 cup white rice, cooked
- ½ cup corn
- A pinch of salt and black pepper
- 2 colored bell peppers, tops, and insides scooped out
- ½ cup tomato sauce

Directions:

1. In a bowl, mix the onion with the oil, paprika, and the other ingredients except for the peppers and tomato sauce, stir well and stuff the peppers with this mix.

2. Put the peppers in the slow cooker, add the sauce, put the lid on, and cook on Low for 4 hours.

3. Transfer the peppers to a platter and serve as an appetizer.

Nutrition: calories 309, fat 188, carbs 3, protein 18

Corn Dip

Preparation time: *10 minutes*

Cooking time: *2 hours*

Servings: *2*

Ingredients:

- 1 cup corn
- 1 tablespoon chives, chopped
- ½ cup heavy cream
- 2 ounces cream cheese, cubed
- ¼ teaspoon chili powder

Directions:

1. In your slow cooker, mix the corn with the chives and the other ingredients, whisk, put the lid on and cook on Low for 2 hours.

2. Divide into bowls and serve as a dip.

Nutrition: calories 123, fat 3, carbs 2, protein 6

CHAPTER 13:

Optavia Appetizer Recipes

Salmon Burger

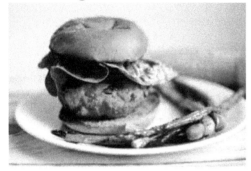

Preparation Time: 15 minutes

Cooking Time: 15 minutes

Servings: 6

Ingredients:

- 16 ounces (450 g) pink salmon, minced
- 1 cup (250 g) prepared mashed potatoes
- 1 medium (110 g) onion, chopped
- 1 stalk celery (about 60 g), finely chopped
- 1 large egg (about 60 g), lightly beaten
- 2 tablespoons (7 g) fresh cilantro, chopped
- 1 cup (100 g) breadcrumbs
- Vegetable oil, for deep frying
- Salt and freshly ground black pepper

Directions:

1. Combine the salmon, mashed potatoes, onion, celery, egg, and cilantro in a mixing bowl. Season to taste and mix thoroughly. Spoon about 2 Tablespoon mixture, roll in breadcrumbs, and then form into small patties.

2. Heat oil in non-stick frying pan. Cook your salmon patties for 5 minutes on each side or until golden brown and crispy.

3. Serve in burger buns and with coleslaw on the side if desired.

Nutrition: calories 230, Fat 7, Carbs 20, Protein 18

Salmon Sandwich with Avocado and Egg

Preparation Time: 15 minutes

Cooking Time: 10 minutes

Servings: 4

Ingredients:

- 8 ounces (250 g) smoked salmon, thinly sliced
- 1 medium (200 g) ripe avocado, thinly sliced
- 4 large poached eggs (about 60 g each)
- 4 slices whole wheat bread (about 30 g each)
- 2 cups (60 g) arugula or baby rocket
- Salt and freshly ground black pepper

Directions:

1. Place 1 bread slice on a plate top with arugula, avocado, salmon, and poached egg. Season with salt and pepper. Repeat the procedure for the remaining ingredients.

2. Serve and enjoy.

Nutrition: calories 310, fat 18, carbs 7, protein 12

Spinach and Cottage Cheese Sandwich

Preparation Time: *15 minutes*

Cooking Time: *10 minutes*

Servings: 4

Ingredients:

- 4 ounces (125 g) cottage cheese
- 1/4 cup (15 g) chives, chopped
- 1 teaspoon (5 g) capers
- 1/2 teaspoon (2.5 g) grated lemon rind
- 4 (2 oz. or 60 g) smoked salmon
- 2 cups (60 g) loose baby spinach
- 1 medium (110 g) red onion, sliced thinly
- 8 slices rye bread (about 30 g each)
- Kosher salt and freshly ground black pepper

Directions:

1. Preheat your griddle or Panini press.
2. Mix together cottage cheese, chives, capers, and lemon rind in a small bowl.
3. Spread and divide the cheese mixture on 4 bread slices. Top with spinach, onion slices, and smoked salmon.
4. Cover with remaining bread slices.
5. Grill the sandwiches until golden and grill marks form on both sides.
6. Transfer to a serving dish.
7. Serve and enjoy.

Nutrition: calories 386, fat 1, carbs 18, protein 1

Feta and Pesto Wrap

Preparation Time: 15 minutes

Cooking Time: 10 minutes

Servings: 4

Ingredients:

- 8 ounces (250 g) smoked salmon fillet, thinly sliced
- 1 cup (150 g) feta cheese
- 8 (15 g) Romaine lettuce leaves
- 4 (6-inch) pita bread
- 1/4 cup (60 g) basil pesto sauce

Directions:

1. Place 1 pita bread on a plate. Top with lettuce, salmon, feta cheese, and pesto sauce. Fold or roll to enclose filling. Repeat the procedure for the remaining ingredients.
2. Serve and enjoy.

Nutrition: calories 408, fat 2, carbs 1, protein 11

Cheese and Onion on Bagel

Preparation Time: 15 minutes

Cooking Time: 10 minutes

Servings: 4

Ingredients:

- 8 ounces (250 g) smoked salmon fillet, thinly sliced
- 1/2 cup (125 g) cream cheese
- 1 medium (110 g) onion, thinly sliced
- 4 bagels (about 80g each), split
- 2 tablespoons (7 g) fresh parsley, chopped
- Freshly ground black pepper to taste

Directions:

1. Spread the cream cheese on each bottom's half of bagels. Top with salmon and onion, season with pepper, sprinkle with parsley, and then cover with bagel tops.
2. Serve and enjoy.

Nutrition:

Calories: 34

Carbs: 0g

Fat: 1g

Protein: 5g

Greek Baklava

Preparation Time: *20 minutes*
Cooking Time: *20 minutes*
Servings: 18
Ingredients:

- 1 (16 oz.) package phyllo dough
- 1 lb. chopped nuts
- 1 cup butter
- 1 teaspoon ground cinnamon
- 1 cup water
- 1 cup white sugar
- 1 teaspoon. vanilla extract
- 1/2 cup honey

Directions:

1. Preheat the oven to 175°C or 350°Fahrenheit. Spread butter on the sides and bottom of a 9-in by 13-in pan.
2. Chop the nuts, then mix with cinnamon; set it aside. Unfurl the phyllo dough, then halve the whole stack to fit the pan. Use a damp cloth to cover the phyllo to prevent drying as you proceed. Put two phyllo sheets in the pan, then butter well. Repeat to make eight layered phyllo sheets. Scatter 2-3 tablespoons. nut mixture over the sheets, then place two more phyllo sheets on top, butter, then sprinkle with nuts. Layer as you go. The final layer should be six to eight phyllo sheets deep.
3. Make square or diamond shapes with a sharp knife up to the bottom of the pan. You can slice into four long rows for diagonal shapes. Bake until crisp and golden for 50 minutes.
4. Meanwhile, boil water and sugar until the sugar melts to make the sauce; mix in honey and vanilla. Let it simmer for 20 minutes.
5. Take the baklava out of the oven, then drizzle with sauce right away; cool. Serve the baklava in cupcake papers.

You can also freeze them without cover. The baklava will turn soggy when wrapped.

Nutrition: Calories: 255 Fat: 15g Saturated Fat: 4g Trans Fat: 0g Cholesterol: 14g Fiber: 2g Sodium: 403mg Protein: 25g

Bananas in Nut Cups

Preparation Time: 30 minutes
Cooking Time: 45 minutes
Servings: 6 servings
Ingredients:

- 3/4 cup shelled pistachios
- 1/2 cup sugar
- 1 teaspoon. ground cinnamon
- 4 sheets phyllo dough, (14 inches x 9 inches) - 1/4 cup butter, melted

Sauce:

- 3/4 cup butter, cubed
- 3/4 cup packed brown sugar
- 3 medium firm bananas, sliced
- 1/4 teaspoon. ground cinnamon
- 3 to 4 cups vanilla ice cream

Directions:

1. Finely chop sugar and pistachios in a food processor; move to a bowl, then mix in cinnamon. Slice each phyllo sheet into 6 four-inch squares, get rid of the trimmings. Pile the squares, then use plastic wrap to cover.
2. Pile 3 squares, flip each at an angle to misalign the corners. Force each stack on the sides and bottom of an oiled eight-oz. custard cup. Bake for 15-20 minutes in a 350 degrees F oven until golden; cool for 5 minutes. Move to a wire rack to cool completely.
3. Melt and boil brown sugar and butter in a saucepan to make the sauce; lower heat. Mix in cinnamon and bananas gently; heat completely. Put ice cream

in the phyllo cups until full, then put banana sauce on top. Serve right away.

Nutrition: calories 100, fat 12, carbs 2, protein 4

Apple Salad Sandwich

Preparation Time: 15 minutes

Cooking Time: 10 minutes

Servings: 4

Ingredients:

- 4 ounces (125 g) canned pink salmon, drained and flaked
- 1 medium (180 g) red apple, cored and diced
- 1 celery stalk (about 60 g), chopped
- 1 shallot (about 40 g), finely chopped
- 1/3 cup (85 g) light mayonnaise
- 8 slices whole grain bread (about 30 g each), toasted
- 8 (15 g) Romaine lettuce leaves
- Salt and freshly ground black pepper

Directions:

1. Combine the salmon, apple, celery, shallot, and mayonnaise in a mixing bowl. Season with salt and pepper.
2. Place 1 slice of bread on a plate, top with lettuce and salmon salad, and then covers with another slice of bread. Repeat the procedure for the remaining ingredients. Serve and enjoy.

Nutrition: calories 121, fat 1, carbs 18, protein 1

Buttermilk Ice Cream Shake

Preparation Time: 5 minutes

Cooking Time: 0 minutes

Servings: 4

Ingredients:

- 3 cups chilled buttermilk
- 1/2 cup cold lemon juice
- Pinch of salt - 1/2 cup sugar

- 1/8 teaspoon grated lemon zest
- 1 cup vanilla ice cream
- Dash ginger

Directions

1. Blend or shake all of the ingredients. Serve the shake together with the ginger.

Nutrition: calories 332, fat 8, carbs 1, protein 14

Buttermilk Shake

Preparation Time: 5 minutes

Cooking Time: 0 minutes

Servings: 4

Ingredients:

- 1 pint vanilla ice cream
- 1 cup buttermilk
- 1 teaspoon grated lemon zest
- 1/2 teaspoon vanilla extract
- 1 drop lemon extract

Directions

1. In a blender container, combine all the ingredients and process them at high speed until smooth. Pour the drink into the glasses. Make sure to put all the leftovers inside the refrigerator.

Nutrition: calories 309, fat 26, carbs 9, protein 12

Cantaloupe Orange Milk Shakes

Preparation Time: 5 minutes

Cooking Time: 0 minutes

Servings: 4

Ingredients:

- 4-1/2 teaspoons orange juice concentrate
- 3/4 cup cubed cantaloupe
- 1 cup vanilla ice cream or frozen yogurt
- 3/4 cup milk
- 3 tablespoons sugar

Directions

1. Mix cantaloupe and orange juice concentrate in a blender. Cover the blender and process it until smooth. Add the sugar, milk, and ice cream. Cover again and process until well-blended. Pour the mixture into the chilled glasses and serve.

Nutrition: calories 252, fat 9, carbs 2, protein 11

Cheese on Rye Bread

Preparation Time: 15 minutes

Cooking Time: 10 minutes

Servings: 4

Ingredients:

- 8 ounces (250 g) smoked salmon, thinly sliced
- 1/3 cup (85 g) mayonnaise
- 2 tablespoons (30 ml) lemon juice
- 1 tablespoon (15 g) Dijon mustard
- 1 teaspoon (3 g) garlic, minced
- 4 slices cheddar cheese (about 2 oz. or 30 g each)
- 8 slices rye bread (about 2 oz. or 30 g each)
- 8 (15 g) Romaine lettuce leaves
- Salt and freshly ground black pepper

Directions:

1. Mix together the mayonnaise, lemon juice, mustard, and garlic in a small bowl. Flavor with salt and pepper and set aside.
2. Spread dressing on 4 bread slices. Top with lettuce, salmon, and cheese. Cover with remaining rye bread slices.
3. Serve and enjoy.

Nutrition: calories 321, fat 1, carbs 8, protein 5

Bulgur Lamb Meatballs

Preparation Time: 10 minutes

Cooking Time: 15 minute

Servings: 6

Ingredients:

- 1 and ½ cups Greek yogurt
- ½ teaspoon cumin, ground
- 1 cup cucumber, shredded
- ½ teaspoon garlic, minced
- A pinch of salt and black pepper
- 1 cup bulgur - 2 cups water
- 1 pound lamb, ground
- ¼ cup parsley, chopped
- ¼ cup shallots, chopped
- ½ teaspoon allspice, ground
- ½ teaspoon cinnamon powder
- 1 tablespoon olive oil

Directions:

1. In a bowl, combine the bulgur with the water, cover the bowl, leave aside for 10 minutes, drain and transfer to a bowl.
2. Add the meat, the yogurt, and the rest of the ingredients except the oil, stir well and shape medium meatballs out of this mix.
3. Heat up a pan with the oil over medium-high heat, add the meatballs, cook them for 7 minutes on each side, arrange them all on a platter and serve as an appetizer.

Nutrition: calories 226, fat 2, carbs 1, protein 3

Cucumber Bites

Preparation Time: 10 minutes

Cooking Time: 0 minutes

Servings: 12

Ingredients:

- 1 English cucumber, sliced into 32 rounds - 10 ounces hummus

- 16 cherry tomatoes, halved
- 1 tablespoon parsley, chopped
- 1 ounce feta cheese, crumbled

Directions:

1. Spread the hummus on each cucumber round, divide the tomato halves on each, sprinkle the cheese and parsley on to, and serve as an appetizer.

Nutrition: calories 209, fat 2, carbs 4, protein 2

241. Hummus with Ground Lamb

Preparation Time: 10 minutes

Cooking Time: 15 minute

Servings: 8

Ingredients:

- 10 ounces hummus
- 12 ounces lamb meat, ground
- ½ cup pomegranate seeds
- ¼ cup parsley, chopped
- 1 tablespoon olive oil
- Pita chips for serving

Directions:

1. Heat up a pan with the oil over medium-high heat, add the meat, and brown for 15 minutes stirring often.
2. Spread the hummus on a platter, spread the ground lamb all over, also spread the pomegranate seeds and the parsley, and serve with pita chips as a snack.

Nutrition: calories 320, fat 2, carbs 1, protein 11

Wrapped Plums

Preparation Time: 5 minutes

Cooking Time: 0 minutes

Servings: 8

Ingredients:

- 2 ounces prosciutto, cut into 16 pieces
- 4 plums, quartered
- 1 tablespoon chives, chopped
- A pinch of red pepper flakes, crushed

Directions:

1. Wrap each plum quarter

Nutrition: calories 209, fat 8, carbs 4, protein 4

Buckwheat Granola

Preparation Time: 15 minutes

Cooking Time: 30 minutes

Servings: 10

Ingredients:

- 2 cups raw buckwheat groats
- ¾ cup pumpkin seeds
- ¾ cup almonds, chopped
- 1 cup unsweetened coconut flakes
- 1 teaspoon ground cinnamon
- 1 teaspoon ground ginger
- 1 ripe banana, peeled
- 2 tablespoons maple syrup
- 2 tablespoons olive oil

Directions:

1. Preheat your oven to 350°F. In a bowl, place the buckwheat groats, coconut flakes, pumpkin seeds, almonds, and spices, and mix well.
2. In another bowl, add the banana, and with a fork, mash well.
3. Add to the buckwheat mixture maple syrup and oil, and mix until well combined.
4. Transfer the mixture onto the prepared baking sheet and spread in an even layer. Bake for about 25–30 minutes, stirring once halfway through.
5. Remove the baking sheet from the oven and set aside to cool.

Nutrition: calories 342, fat 7, carbs 8, protein 10

Apple Pancakes

Preparation Time: 15 minutes
Cooking Time: 24 minutes
Servings: 6
Ingredients:

- ½ cup buckwheat flour
- 2 tablespoons coconut sugar
- 1 teaspoon baking powder
- ½ teaspoon ground cinnamon
- 1/3 cup unsweetened almond milk
- 1 egg, beaten lightly
- 2 granny smith apples, peeled, cored, and grated

Directions:

1. In a bowl, place the flour, coconut sugar, and cinnamon, and mix well.
2. In another bowl, place the almond milk and egg and beat until well combined.
3. Now, place the flour mixture and mix until well combined.
4. Fold in the grated apples.
5. Cook for 1–2 minutes on each side.
6. Repeat with the remaining mixture.
7. Serve warm with the drizzling of honey.

Nutrition: calories 588, fat 3, carbs 8, protein 20

Matcha Pancakes

Preparation Time: 10 minutes
Cooking Time: 25 minutes
Servings: 6
Ingredients:

- 1 cup spelt flour
- 1 cup buckwheat flour
- 1 tablespoon matcha powder
- 1 tablespoon baking powder
- Pinch of salt
- ¾ cup unsweetened almond milk
- 1 tablespoon olive oil
- 1/3 cup raw honey

Directions:

1. In a bowl, add the flax meal and warm water and mix well. Set aside for about 5 minutes.
2. Now, place the flour mixture and mix until a smooth textured mixture is formed.
3. Cook for about 2–3 minutes.
4. Carefully flip the side and cook for about 1 minute.
5. Repeat with the remaining mixture.
6. Serve warm with the drizzling of honey.

Nutrition: calories 345, fat 12, carbs 4, protein 11

Smoked Salmon & Kale Scramble

Preparation Time: 10 minutes
Cooking Time: 9 minutes
Servings: 3
Ingredients:

- 2 cups fresh kale, tough ribs removed and chopped finely
- 1 tablespoon coconut oil
- Ground black pepper to taste
- ½ cup smoked salmon, crumbled
- 4 eggs, beaten

Directions:

1. In a wok, melt the coconut oil over high heat and cook the kale with black pepper for about 3–4 minutes.
2. Stir in the smoked salmon and reduce the heat to medium.
3. Add the eggs and cook for about 3–4 minutes, stirring frequently.
4. Serve immediately.

Nutrition: calories 568, fat 3, carbs 5, protein 10

Kale & Mushroom Frittata

Preparation Time: 15 minutes
Cooking Time: 30 minutes
Servings: 5
Ingredients:

- 8 eggs
- ½ cup unsweetened almond milk
- Salt and ground black pepper to taste
- 1 tablespoon olive oil
- 1 onion, chopped
- 1 garlic clove, minced
- 1 cup fresh mushrooms, chopped
- 1½ cups fresh kale, tough ribs removed and chopped

Directions:

1. Preheat oven to 350°F.
2. In a large bowl, place the eggs, coconut milk, salt, and black pepper, and beat well. Set aside.
3. In a large ovenproof wok, heat the oil over medium heat and sauté the onion and garlic for about 3–4 minutes.
4. Add the squash, kale, bell pepper, salt, and black pepper, and cook for about 8–10 minutes.
5. Stir in the mushrooms and cook for about 3–4 minutes.
6. Add the kale and cook for about 5 minutes.
7. Place the egg mixture on top evenly and cook for about 4 minutes, without stirring.
8. Transfer the wok to the oven and bake for about 12–15 minutes or until desired doneness.
9. Remove from the oven and place the frittata side for about 3–5 minutes before serving. Cut into desired sized wedges and serve.

Nutrition: calories 356, fat 2, carbs 4, protein 8

Kale, Apple, & Cranberry Salad

Preparation Time: 15 minutes
Cooking Time: 15 minutes
Servings: 4
Ingredients:

- 6 cups fresh baby kale
- 3 large apples, cored and sliced
- ¼ cup unsweetened dried cranberries
- ¼ cup almonds, sliced
- 2 tablespoons extra-virgin olive oil
- 1 tablespoon raw honey
- Salt and ground black pepper to taste

Directions:

1. In a salad bowl, place all the ingredients and toss to coat well.
2. Serve immediately.

Nutrition: calories 209, fat 2, carbs 5, protein 8

Arugula, Strawberry, & Orange Salad

Preparation Time: 15 minutes
Cooking Time: 15 minutes
Servings: 4
Ingredients:
Salad

- 6 cups fresh baby arugula
- 1½ cups fresh strawberries, hulled and sliced
- 2 oranges, peeled and segmented

Dressing

- 2 tablespoons fresh lemon juice
- 1 tablespoon raw honey
- 2 teaspoons extra-virgin olive oil
- 1 teaspoon Dijon mustard
- Salt and ground black pepper to taste

Directions:

1. For salad: in a salad bowl, place all ingredients and mix.

2. For dressing: place all ingredients in another bowl and beat until well combined.
3. Place dressing on top of the salad and toss to coat well.
4. Serve immediately.

Nutrition: calories 389, fat 8, carbs 4, protein 7

Lean and Green Crockpot Chili

Preparation Time: 3 minutes

Cooking Time: 45 minutes

Servings: 8

Ingredients:

- 1-pound boneless skinless chicken breasts, cut into strips
- ½ cup chopped onion
- 2 teaspoons ground cumin
- 1 teaspoon minced garlic
- ½ teaspoon chili powder
- Salt and pepper to taste
- 1 ½ cups water
- 1 can green enchilada sauce
- ½ cup dried beans, soaked overnight

Directions:

1. Place all ingredients in a pot.
2. Mix all ingredients until combined.
3. Close the lid and turn on the heat to medium.
4. Bring to a boil and allow to simmer for 45 minutes or until the beans are cooked.
5. Serve with chopped cilantro on top.

Nutrition: Calories: 84; Protein: 13.4g; Carbs: 3.6 g; Fat: 1.7g Sugar: 0.8g

Conclusion

When you desire a structure and need to rapidly lose weight, the optavia diet is the perfect solution.

The extremely low calories eating plans of the optavia diet will definitely help you to shed more pounds

Before you start any meal replacement diet plan, carefully consider if truly it possible for you to continue with a specific diet plan

When you have decided to stick with optavia and make progress with your weight loss goal, ensure you have a brilliant knowledge about optimal health management to enable and archive the desired result effortlessly in the shortest period of time.

CPSIA information can be obtained
at www.ICGtesting.com
Printed in the USA
LVHW070126210221
679537LV00037B/1642